Praise for *Mindfulness: A Kindly Approach to Being with Cancer*

A diagnosis of cancer can produce waves of shock, confusion and despair affecting not only the sufferer, but also family and close friends. Where can you turn? What resources can you find right now that will ease the pain? From start to finish, Trish Bartley provides the best sort of support for anyone suffering such anguish. Drawing on her own experience of recurrent cancer and using her long and deep experience as international mindfulness teacher and trainer, she offers words you can trust. Here is not only something to read, but something to practice.

Mark Williams,
Emeritus Professor of Clinical Psychology,
Oxford Mindfulness Centre, University of Oxford, UK

How do we skilfully meet suffering with kindness? Trish has distilled her years of experience into this wonderfully clear and accessible guide to mindfulness. An embodiment of compassion and wisdom, and an inspiring read.

Rebecca Crane,
Director, Centre for Mindfulness Research and Practice,
Bangor University, UK

Trish has distilled the very essence of Mindfulness in a way that makes it accessible for folks who may be at the most stressful time of their life. All of us experience pain and fear with physical challenges, and cancer tops the list. What a gentle, useful guidebook for us all and particularly for those handling this big challenge. Thank you, Trish!

Pam Erdmann,
MBSR Teacher, Center for Mindfulness,
University of Massachusetts Medical School, USA

Through the vehicle of mindfulness Trish Bartley is reaching for you. Grab her hand. It will light a fire in the face of fear. Become a warrior for gentleness. Medicine needs this book. We all need this book.

Dr. Anna Mandeville,
Consultant Clinical Health Psychologist

This is a lovely book - wise, compassionate, and very practical. Here is a wonderful friendly guide to tried and tested ways to live more fully and kindly with cancer.

John Teasdale,
Research Scientist, Medical Research Council, Cambridge, UK,
- and author of Affect, Cognition, and Change and Mindfulness-based
Cognitive Therapy for Depression

Mindfulness: A Kindly Approach to Being with Cancer

Trish Bartley

WILEY Blackwell

This edition first published 2017
© 2017 John Wiley & Sons, Ltd

Registered Office
John Wiley & Sons, Ltd, The Atrium, Southern Gate, Chichester, West Sussex, PO19 8SQ, UK

Editorial Offices
350 Main Street, Malden, MA 02148-5020, USA
9600 Garsington Road, Oxford, OX4 2DQ, UK
The Atrium, Southern Gate, Chichester, West Sussex, PO19 8SQ, UK

For details of our global editorial offices, for customer services, and for information about how to apply for permission to reuse the copyright material in this book please see our website at www.wiley.com/wiley-blackwell.

Library of Congress Cataloging-in-Publication data applied for

Hardback ISBN: 9781118926277
Paperback ISBN: 9781118926284

A catalogue record for this book is available from the British Library.

Set in 10/12.5pt Times by SPi Global, Pondicherry, India

Printed in the UK

To the memory of
Christopher, Peggy and Charles,
with my gratitude.

To Eleni, Aris, Elizabeth and Alexander
with my love.

This book is dedicated to helping people with cancer
and other life threatening illness bring
mindfulness and kindness
into their lives.

Also by Trish Bartley

Holding Up the Sky: Love, Power and Learning
in the Development of a Community

Mindfulness-Based Cognitive Therapy for Cancer:
Gently Turning Towards

Contents

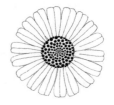

Contents

Acknowledgments

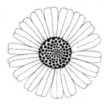

I am very grateful to all those who have helped in many different ways to bring this book into being.

I wish to express particular appreciation to Sarah, Caroline, Peter, Jane and Helen, for their courage, dignity and generosity in being willing to share their stories. I also want to thank all those who wrote poems – almost all of them poetry 'novices', and to all the 'cancer' mindfulness participants who attended classes or worked with me one-to-one, who were willing for their experience to be included in this book. Their motivation to benefit others is inspiring.

Grateful thanks also go to people within Wiley Blackwell and connected to it, who have supported the production of this book. I especially want to thank Andy Peart, Karen Shield and Kathy Syplywczak. Several people have contributed to the illustrations in this book. I am very grateful to Maria Hayes for her beautiful drawings.

Thanks also go to Julie Louwman, Evan Herbert, and Katie Green – and to Stewart Mercer, Jill Teague, Joanna Macy and Anita Burrows for generously allowing me to reproduce their poems.

I am lucky in my colleagues and want to thank them for their support in the writing and shaping of this book. Christina Shennan has read several drafts and been unstinting in her support and wise feedback. Her considerable experience as a teacher and trainer of this approach and her kindly realism has enriched this book. I am also very grateful to those who have given support and feedback especially Jane Maitland, Rebecca Crane, Ursula Bates, Helen Jones and Stirling Moorey. I have much appreciated their wisdom and experience.

I also want to acknowledge the kindness and support of Jody Mardula, Cindy Cooper, Mariel Jones, Janne Foster, Evan and Delphine Herbert, Josephine Seccombe, Diana and Jim Allanson, Ciaran Saunders, David Shannon, Maura Kenny, Davine Thaw, Loretta van Schalkwyk, Nick Stuart, Cath Bale, and the team in Alaw – and many others including Centre for Mindfulness Research and Practice colleagues and friends at Bangor University – and students, trainees and supervisees. They have offered me much learning.

It has not been possible to adequately acknowledge in the notes the particular contribution that Christina Feldman has made to so much of this book. She has been patient, wise and generous. I am especially grateful to her.

I am indebted to all my teachers and mentors, who directly or indirectly offered their guidance, wisdom and inspiration, recently or in the past – in particular Jon Kabat-Zinn and John Teasdale. I also wish to thank Tina Usherwood, Mark Williams, the late Francis Batten, Christina Feldman, Linda Gwillim, Andrew Patching, Ferris Urbanowski, Akincano Marc Weber, Stephen Batchelor, Rigdzin Shikpo and Ken and Elizabeth Mellor.

I am very grateful to my family for their love and support. I dedicate this book with much gratitude to my parents and my brother, who shaped much of my childhood; and with much joy to my four grandchildren, who shape my old age.

About the Companion Website

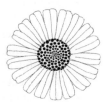

This book is accompanied by a companion website:

www.wiley.com/go/bartley/mindfulness

The website includes:
Mindfulness Practices and Exercises organized around the four key chapters:

1 **Intention**
   - Intentions Practice
   - The Raisin Exercise
   - The Pause (short practice)
   - Feet on the Floor (short practice)
   - Body Scan (core practice)
   - First Aid Practice (cancer practice)

2 **Coming back**
   - Mindful Walking (core practice)
   - Standing in Mountain (short practice)
   - Coming to the Breath (short practice)

- Walking Down the Street Exercise
- Mindful Waiting Practice (cancer practice)
- Two additional Waiting Practices
  - Waiting and breathing with
  - Waiting with kindness
- Mindful Treatment Practice (cancer practice)
- Treatment with Kindness (additional practice)
- Two additional Treatment Practices (combined)
  - Treatment with blessing
  - Treatment and visualization
- Mindful Stretching/Movement Practice (additional core practice)

3 **Turning towards**
- Sitting Practice (core practice)
- The Body Barometer (short practice)
- A Breathing Space (short practice)
- A Mindful Practice for Uncertainty/Breathing Space (cancer practice)

4 **Kindness**
- Walking with Kindness (core practice)
- Coming to the Breath with Kindness (short practice)
- A Three Step Responding Space (short practice)
- The Thread Exercises (cancer practices)

 The easiest way to download the practice materials is onto your computer. Go to the book's website; click on the download link of the file you need; it will save into the downloads folder on your computer. It may also offer you the option to save it where you want it (music folder, etc). When you have it safely on your computer, open it by double clicking on the file. It will play the practice for you through your computer speakers.

If you want to save it onto a tablet or phone, and you are not sure how - ask a teenager for help!

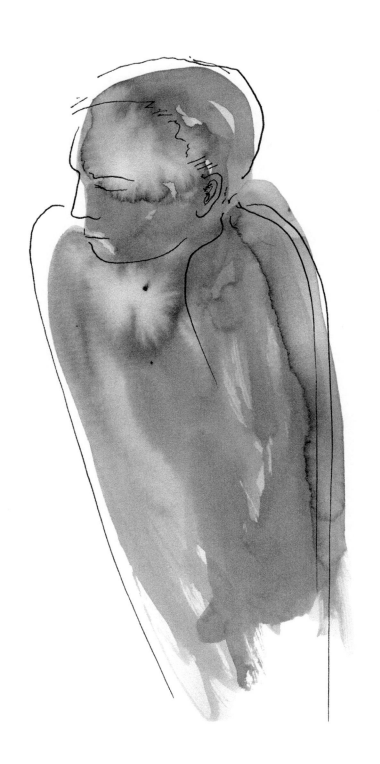

Some Opening Words

Two questions have informed my writing.

What really matters?

What enables us to meet suffering with kindness?

When I was first diagnosed with cancer in 1999, I threw away my diary, for there was little chance of working that year. At the time, this seemed huge. I had been working with people and their struggles for over 25 years. It seemed a part of who I was, what I did. Later I realized, when I sat waiting for treatment that I had never been closer to people in their distress. Here they were – and here I was, one of them.

Two earlier life events had produced a similar crumbling. At the worst of these times, I came to know a sense of groundlessness as an empty sensation deep inside. It would be there on waking, even before my eyes were open. Of course, in time the ground returns and meaning gets cobbled together again. Not even deep distress endures. It morphs, changes shape, puts on new clothes and grows in different directions.

Working with people with cancer asks me to re-visit that place. It is not the same as when tipped into it myself, but I know it well enough to connect with others who are there and not be afraid. Their stories of loss, shock, and fear are all individual and personal, yet we are able to acknowledge the suffering we share. Wherever they are in their experience

Mindfulness: A Kindly Approach to Being with Cancer, First Edition. Trish Bartley.
© 2017 John Wiley & Sons, Ltd. Published 2017 by John Wiley & Sons, Ltd.
Companion Website: www.wiley.com/go/bartley/mindfulness

of cancer, we connect at the beginning of their mindfulness path. With luck, some early threads of trust start weaving that help them learn about being present to their experience.

So, what is it that really matters?

Maybe it is not the suffering, nor the cancer – and not even mindfulness.

Rumi wrote some words that speak of this.

Out beyond ideas of wrong doing and right doing, there is a field. I'll meet you there[1].

This theme runs through this book. How can we meet ourselves in our distress? Deep suffering touches us all eventually. Maybe it is only then that these questions make much sense – for it does not seem to matter whether the meeting is with self or with other. The same quality of kindly attention is called for.

So what of my 'meeting' with you who are reading this? I would love that sense of you to be strong and clear as I write. Many of the people I've taught, walk onto my computer screen, arrive in my memory, remind me of some remark they made, or some experience or insight they shared.

I have sought to hold you, the one who reads, in my heart and mind as I write – linking you to those others I've known and taught. At times, this sense of you fades – and then my confidence dips, washed by doubt, sapping intention. When I feel that, I bring you back to mind – and we journey on together once more. Perhaps you can do the same, connecting with me and with others like you, who are reading as you do.

As I write this, I remember the group of people with cancer who I am currently teaching, in a room off the hospital oncology corridor. As with all groups at the start, I wonder what they will find as they learn to bring mindfulness into their lives. This is the group that will now influence my writing. This is the group that you, my other group, will sit within. Stay in touch as we take this ride together – for it is only in kindly connection that we may discover what really matters to us – and then thread it into our lives.

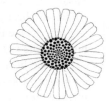

Starting Out

As you unfold, just keep on quietly and earnestly, growing through all that happens to you. You cannot disrupt the process more violently than by looking outside yourself for answers that may only be found by attending to your innermost feeling.

Rainer Maria Rilke[2]

Introduction

Sometimes, certain moments in our lives seem to be freeze framed, as if caught in a spotlight of significance. All that follows becomes 'after'. Getting a cancer diagnosis can be like that – defined by the shock of its impact. Nothing may ever be quite so certain again.

This book is written for people with cancer – or those who have had cancer – who want to find ways of managing their reactions to illness. Whether you already have a mindfulness practice or are interested in developing one, mindfulness can offer you a way of relating differently with what you struggle with. The difficulties will not necessarily go away, but by being with them more gently, things may feel easier and steadier. With practice, dedication and a certain effort, you can cultivate ways of living mindfully, even in the context of anxiety and loss.

Susan was close to retirement when told she had breast cancer. She soldiered through treatment, keeping up a brave face – but at night she raged. One time in bed, she beat her fists onto the mattress and cried bitterly. She felt so wild and furious.

She had been depressed in the past and knew the warning signs – so on hearing about mindfulness from her oncology nurse, Susan expressed interest straightaway. She met others in the same boat and it felt alright to learn mindfulness alongside them. Their reactions were very similar to hers. This helped her come to terms with some of her demons. 'I just went in at the beginning open-minded, thinking I'll suck it and see, and in the end I got myself back – maybe even better'.

A general introduction

This chapter explains how to get the most from this book. By the end of it, I hope you will have a sense of what to expect – and understand that although this approach is carefully structured, you will always be encouraged to find your own way and make your own choices.

This is not a book to 'master', nor is mindfulness an approach to perfect. Instead, we learn to cultivate, develop, and grow mindfulness – like carefully planting a seed that puts down strong roots. This approach invites you to learn from your own experience – listening, reflecting and finding out what feels best for you.

There is no need to be busy with this. It is important to trust your own ways of learning – to adapt things to suit your own style and context, culture and situation. Nor is it to suggest that no effort is needed. For certainly, to cultivate a mindfulness practice that can reliably support you through the ups and downs of life – considerable effort is called for. However, the effort needed is one of gentle persistence, remembering that small steps taken every day are wiser and more sustainable than big ones now and then.

Mindfulness-Based Approaches

Mindfulness is practiced by millions of people who stop and come back to their direct experience *now*, maybe for some minutes – maybe only for a moment or two. By doing this, they develop the possibility of cultivating a more skilful and kindly way of being.

Evidence of the benefit of mindfulness-based approaches is growing steadily – for people with general challenges (such as stress), and also for those with specific conditions (such as depression, anxiety and cancer[3]). This approach has something universal to offer, whatever life circumstance we find ourselves in. Specific mindfulness-based programs have been adapted to the needs of particular populations, such as this one for people with cancer – although the approach we take in this book will have many resonances for people experiencing a range of different challenges.

Background to mindfulness-based approaches

In the 1980s, Jon Kabat-Zinn developed eight-week mindfulness-based courses[4], in a Massachusetts university hospital, for people with a wide range of different conditions and everyday life challenges. He called his program Mindfulness-Based Stress Reduction – MBSR for short.

The foundation of the program brought together a number of significant influences including early contemplative Buddhist practice and Western psychological understanding of suffering. However, Jon has been clear from the beginning that MBSR is secular. It needs to be accessible and relevant to people from all traditions and none. Jon's genius lies in the foundations of the program itself; its accessibility to ordinary people; and in the clarity, values and wisdom that underpin it.

MBSR started a worldwide development. It has transformed what is now available to support human flourishing and well-being. It is taught in diverse contexts such as education, health, criminal justice, and the workplace. All the many mindfulness-based developments that have emerged are based on MBSR – the grandmother and grandfather of them all.

Mindfulness-based cognitive therapy for depression

An early development took place in the UK and Canada, which was led by three distinguished psychologists, working in the field of recurrent depression. John Teasdale, Mark Williams and Zindel Segal developed Mindfulness-Based Cognitive Therapy for Depression[5], known as MBCT. It was found to nearly halve the risk of relapse in participants with three or more previous episodes of depression. This MBCT research established a new standard in evidence for the effectiveness of mindfulness-based approaches. Many randomised control trials researching MBCT have followed which replicate this first finding, and extend the evidence to new contexts and populations. The most compelling endorsement for MBCT comes from the UK's National Institute for Health and Care Excellence (NICE), which provides clinical guidelines for evidence-based care. NICE have consistently recommended MBCT since 2004 for people who are vulnerable to repeated depression.

Mindfulness-based cognitive therapy for people with cancer

In this book, we explore mindfulness through the building blocks of a program that was developed in the UK, specifically for people with cancer. Mindfulness-Based Cognitive Therapy for Cancer[6] was adapted directly from MBCT for Depression, which in turn comes out of MBSR.

I developed MBCT for Cancer (MBCT-Ca for short) with a lot of support from teaching and medical colleagues, over many years in a hospital oncology department in North Wales. It has now been taught to people with all types and stages of cancer in many different hospital and community settings in the UK, Europe and further afield.

I was lucky to be amongst an early group of people who were trained by Jon Kabat-Zinn and others in the UK, around the time that the first MBCT research trial was reporting its findings. I had just finished my own treatment and decided to teach MBCT to others with cancer. Two of the original founders of MBCT, Mark Williams and John Teasdale, supported and guided me in developing this work.

Ten years later, I was diagnosed with another cancer as I was writing up *MBCT for Cancer*, aimed at teachers.[5] Now, some years later and happily in good health, I write this book for people with cancer themselves. It draws on the experience of hundreds of people who have followed the program; on feedback from close colleagues who have taught it; and on my own understanding through teaching patients, training teachers and using MBCT-Ca in my own experience of cancer.

The approach in this book is very similar to that program, but follows a different time frame. This allows you to take as long as you want with each section. You can find your own pace and rhythm, and mould your learning to suit your context and personal situation.

The Structure of the Book

We follow a similar format in each chapter. I will list the key ingredients and then describe them in a bit more detail.

There are three sections in each chapter:

1 *Theme* – the first section develops your understanding of the key theme of the chapter. They are based on four 'movements' of mindful awareness.
2 *Practices and exercises/approaches* – the second explores mindfulness as a practice – both through a core practice (which builds the momentum of mindfulness) and through short practices woven into your day (so that they are accessible to you whenever you need them). The practices are available on the book's website for you to download. We also look at ways of better understanding the habitual patterns of mind.
3 *The experience of cancer* – the last section considers the impact of cancer at various points, (diagnosis, treatment, etc.) and suggests some targeted practices. People with cancer share ways they find to resource themselves.

Woven through the book are poems and personal stories by people with cancer, who practice mindfulness. They form the heart of this book and accompany you through every page.

1   The themes – four movements of mindfulness

Bringing mindfulness into your life is a radical way of being with cancer. Our tendency is to dwell on things that *might* happen in the future, or that *have* happened in the past. We get sucked into believing the stories that get played out in the mind. Instead, with kindly patience and mindful practice, we learn to come back to focus on our present moment experience.

This may not sound radical, but when we manage to respond in this way, we are changing the habits of a lifetime. We learn to recognise that the way the mind reacts often *adds* to what is already difficult. We start to find another place to stand – anchored in the immediacy of our felt experience, *now*.

We will still be affected by difficulty – of course. Like trees in a storm, there is no escaping the wildness of the weather at times. Yet when the wind abates, the trees return to stillness. Those that survive the best, have roots that go deep, and trunks that flex and bend. They do not try to resist or fight the wind, as we tend to.

Each of us, who has had a cancer diagnosis, has times of feeling blown about by strong feelings – fear, sadness, anger, or any combination. The force of these 'storms' varies – just like the strength of the wind – but by putting down roots that offer stability, and learning to be gentle with ourselves in the midst of intensity – the strength and duration of the emotions lessen.

With lots of practice, some key understanding and a willingness to bring kindness to the 'weather patterns' of the mind, we can develop tools and skills that help us stay balanced and steady, which allow us to manage things differently.

The four movements, which are set out in this book, offer a pathway into this different way of being with cancer. Like all significant journeys, we never quite know where we will end up – but walking with courage, kindness and curiosity as best we can, and connecting with others like us along the way, we can stay open to whatever opportunities it may offer.

Intention is the first step on the path, and though it may seem the least tangible, it may prove to be the most important. It is the way we bring the mind on board as an ally. Intention acts like a compass, or signpost, pointing out the direction we need to take.

Coming Back is next. It is the foundation of mindful awareness practice. We learn to come back, again and again, to be aware of our immediate experience, whatever it is.

Turning Towards is the radical one of the four. We all try to avoid what we do not want – even the simplest organisms do that. We also tend to rush past what we enjoy, especially when times are tough. By practicing 'turning towards' little by little, we start to notice and appreciate what is pleasant, and respond more gently to what is not.

Kindness is there all along, like a soft breeze, befriending practice and experience. It is integral to mindfulness and is how we transform our relationship to our experience.

Here is an example of someone using these four movements:

Rosemary woke with a heavy sense of dread. She had a check-up that afternoon. She remembered her intention to keep connecting with her present experience – so she took a few mindful breaths, before getting out of bed. Throughout the morning, she remembered to keep coming back by feeling the contact of her feet on the floor. She left early for the hospital and met up with a friend. They sat together in the waiting area. Heart pounding, thoughts racing, Rosemary kept remembering her intention. Turning towards the unpleasant sensations in her belly, she breathed with them, holding them gently in awareness, and bringing kindness in on the breath as she had been taught. 'It wasn't pleasant', she told her mother later, 'but it could have been an awful lot worse. My mindfulness practice definitely helped.'

2 Practices and exercises/approaches

In each chapter, you will be introduced to key mindfulness practices. Some of these are referred to as 'core' practices. They last for various amounts of time – never more than 30 minutes and some for considerably less. These core practices are important in building the momentum of mindfulness. They need regular commitment to practice – and we look at ways of developing this throughout the book.

You are guided through the practices with recordings that you can download from the website connected to this book. Part of your preparation for using this book will be to get the practices onto your phone or somewhere easily accessible. We use various symbols to help you navigate through the book. A key to these is included below.

There are also two key short practices in each chapter that are just as important as the 'core' practices. They are brief, sometimes lasting for only a few seconds. They are simple to learn. You are encouraged to practice them during your day, wherever you are, without the use of the recording, once they are familiar to you. They will then be there 'in your back pocket' whenever and wherever you need them, as tools and resources to support you.

There are also some additional practices, designed to deepen the experience for those more familiar with mindfulness. You may find that by learning the key practices first, you will then be able to adapt and develop them – either along the lines suggested, or in your own way.

These first two sections – the themes and the practices – are there to help you build an understanding of the ways that you struggle and how mindfulness can intervene. This two-sided approach of understanding and practice is carried through the book. Mindfulness is often seen as yet another self-help 'technique'. As your experience and understanding grows, you may come to appreciate that it is more helpfully understood as 'a way of being' that can be threaded into everyday life. This has the powerful potential of building your capacity for steadiness and contentment.

3 The experience of cancer

Towards the end of the first four chapters, there is a section that speaks to a different aspect of the experience of cancer. These include a number of specific 'cancer' practices, relevant to different times – such as undergoing treatment, diagnosis, uncertainty, recurrence and so on.

Each of you has your own story of cancer and your own individual process and context. Some of these sections will not apply to you – or they will refer to times long gone. Some may point to your worst dread or connect you to days that were or are very difficult. It is natural to want to push these associations away and put them behind you. However, when the moment feels right, you might want to see if you can use your mindfulness practice to support you to explore what is relevant and helpful.

There are two further chapters after the four 'movement' chapters. One helps you gather your learning and draw up a plan to continue. The final chapter explores themes of interconnection and discusses how to live mindfully in the context of uncertainty.

Travelling With Others

You will read many stories and anecdotes from people much like you. Their names have been changed. All those involved were happy for their experience to be shared, in order to support others like them. Through them, you learn skills and develop tools that will help you manage your days.

There are also five interviews that are called Personal Stories. I am very grateful to these five for being willing to share their experience of cancer and mindfulness. It is a very brave and generous thing to do.

Descriptions of what has been helpful, may also remind you of things that supported you in the past that you can bring back into use again now. The people that you read about will become your teachers and travelling companions. They will connect you to what helps, because they know what it is like.

Having cancer can feel lonely – however kind and supportive family and friends may be. So at times we will make a point of linking with other people also reading this book, who, like you, are practicing mindfulness in the context of cancer. You may never meet any of them – but together we form a community of mindfulness practitioners, by allowing these connections into our hearts to offer a sense of support. In this way, we can help each other keep going when the going gets tough, or when it feels difficult to sustain practice.

How To Get The Most Out Of This Book

Your experience of mindfulness

Some of you may be familiar with mindfulness. Perhaps you were introduced to it through an eight-week course before you were diagnosed. Your practice may be central to how you are managing – or, as is often the case, you may be finding it hard to reconnect with it after experiencing some tough times. This book may be a way back – perhaps to deepen your practice, and to enable you to focus on what mindfulness might offer you in this context of cancer. You may also find it is helpful to use this book alongside an eight-week mindfulness course.

Others of you may be relatively or completely new to mindfulness. Perhaps you have been given this book, or found it yourself, in the hope that it may offer you a new way of accessing support, as you adjust to the implications of living with cancer.

As you go through these chapters, you may find that some of the material may not be relevant until you are a little more experienced in this approach. You may want to return and re-read parts later, when you have established the basics of your practice. I have sought to signpost the sections clearly, often using symbols to help you. These will point out the *key practices* for you to follow. There are others, which we term *additional practices* that will probably be more relevant later to those with more experience. However, the choice is always yours. Mindfulness may be new to you, but some of the additional practices may be the most useful.

Whatever your situation and experience, we seek to build on the existing approaches and practices that you use, and develop and create new ones. The entire focus is for you to discover and put in place what is most helpful.

Your experience of cancer

You will all be at different points in relation to getting cancer. Some of you may come across this book very early, soon after diagnosis. Others may be later down the line. Wherever you are, you will inevitably be drawn to those sections that seem most relevant to the place that you have reached. You will find dedicated practices designed to support you.

It is fine to turn straight to the section that you are drawn to. In your shoes, I probably would. However, it may also be helpful to retrace your tracks and catch up on earlier sections that have led up to that point. This book is carefully planned to build chapter on chapter, practice on practice, along the lines of the eight-week MBSR and MBCT course. It obviously helps to work through from the beginning. The 'cancer' practices are often the same as (or developed out of) the key short practices in the previous section. You cannot hope to integrate these immediately – so it makes sense to learn and practice them in an everyday context, so that when you need them 'in earnest', they will be readily available to you.

Although this particular approach has been specifically developed for you and others with cancer, it is rooted in principles that have been crafted over many years by some of the finest hearts and minds of this and former times.

Navigation signposts

Key Practices	
Core Practice	
Short Practice	
Other recurring symbols	
'Cancer' Practice	
Download available (see Companion Website page for details)	
Reflective inquiry	

Additional practices will not have any special symbols but are clearly named. 'Cancer' Practices use a 'thread', which is explained below – Preparing to Start: Making a Thread. Reflective Inquiry will also come clear to you once you get into the chapters.

Preparing To Start

Practical materials

1 Notebook

Find a notebook that fits a pocket or bag. Have it with you wherever you go with a pen to hand as well. Over time, it can become something to turn to, like a confidante – to record a piece of information; note how you are feeling; the title of some music; a question you want to think about; the snatch of a poem; maybe a sketch.

At the start of this chapter, Rilke encourages us to attend to[7] our innermost feelings. They can take time to get to know. Your notebook may help with this. Let no one see it, not even your closest friend. When we write with the possibility of other eyes looking, the writing changes. Self-consciousness emerges. We then write for who might see, not for the sake of simply expressing what needs to be expressed.

2 Downloading the practices

I was told recently that resource materials are often not downloaded from book websites. My heart sank. I hope you will be different!

I encourage you to download all the practices now before you go much further – or ask someone to do this for you. Decide where you will put them – perhaps on your phone, tablet, or computer. Like your notebook, it is important to have them easily accessible. The practices have been recorded especially for you to use with this program. Without them this book will be of limited use.

3 Making a 'thread'

Another practical task is to make a simple bracelet, known as 'Thought on a Thread'[8]. We use a black cotton thread and a red bead, but you can choose your own colour and material.

The greatest challenge in learning mindfulness is to remember the practices – especially the short ones. Setting up reminders can make all the difference. Wearing a 'thought on a thread' on your wrist nudges you to remember the short practices – and connects you to thousands of other men and women also wearing threads and practicing mindfulness – just like you.

The thread is used with the dedicated 'cancer' practices. Many find they help them remember to 'come back' and be mindful, especially during difficult times.

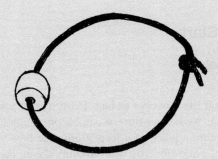

Materials
Thong black cotton (thread) 1.5 mm thick – 12" (30 cm) per bracelet
    Red Wood Barrel Pony (bead) 8 × 10 mm – 1 for each bracelet
Instructions
It could not be simpler. Thread the bead onto the cotton and tie it onto your wrist (your dominant hand is best). Using a reef knot – right over left and left over right – trim the ends and you are done.
    (See www.thoughtonathread.co.uk[7])

You may have friends who want to know what they can do to help. If so, you can ask them to make you a thread or two. If you want to modify the materials, or change the colours, the intention is still the same. You can make threads for your family and friends as a way of staying connected if you need to go into hospital. Children love these and understand the message of connection that they offer.

Beginning Orientation

Here is some general guidance.

Scepticism is welcome!
There is no need to imagine that you have to 'believe' in mindfulness for it to 'work'. Approaching it with curiosity, to see what it offers you – is a good place to start from and continue with.

Learning from experience

Mindfulness is based on experiential learning. It requires us to recognise that we are the experts in our own experience. We can learn a great deal from others, but we benefit from attending to and cultivating our own 'inner wisdom'. This asks you to check things out for yourself, rather than take on anything you are unsure of.

Staying open to outcomes

You may get what you want from this book – but many of us do not know what is possible until we have experienced it. So staying open is a wise option, without expectation or judgement. In this way, you can discern what mindfulness offers you and what choices might work best for you.

Taking each chapter one at a time

We tend to pick up a book and rifle through it looking for the 'juicy' bits. This is how we live life – grazing on the sound bites, quickly judging and moving on. The invitation here is to do it differently. See if you can take your time and savour the parts you enjoy and reflect on those that challenge or surprise you. You can decide not to read ahead to the next chapter, until you are fully ready. It is quite a discipline!

Choosing the best time

When might be a good time for you to start? You may want to reflect on this. If you have a lot going on right now – or you have recently been diagnosed, you might want to dip into parts – using some of the short dedicated cancer practices for example – and then return to work through the sections more methodically later, when things are more manageable.

Invest in your preparation

There are a few things to do before starting. Some are practical and some look at ways of supporting your learning.

Support plans to put in place

Family support It is worth getting your family onside with your plans. There will be times when you are practicing and will not be available – perhaps for up to 30 minutes. They can support you by not interrupting. Younger members of the family might enjoy practicing with you for short periods.

Support person It is helpful to have someone specific to support you. Sometimes, motivation can dip. We need to dig in at these times, and remember why we are doing it – and get help to keep going. It is worth it – for if you give up, you will not be able to maintain what you have learnt, and your time and effort will be wasted.

If there is someone in your life who is interested in mindfulness, and/or would be willing to support you, ask him or her now. Their job is to remind you that there may be times when you feel like giving up – and to see how they can help you keep going. This support may make all the difference between continuing and giving up.

Counsellor Some of you may be receiving professional support. It would certainly be worth telling him or her about your intentions around mindfulness, which they will have heard of and may even be practicing or teaching themselves.

Family, friends, colleagues and health professionals can all offer you invaluable support as you embark on bringing mindfulness into your life. Setting this up in advance is a skilful way of ensuring that you keep your learning going, maintain your intention to support your health and wellbeing, and reap the benefits of living more mindfully.

Understanding The Challenges

There is much potential in embarking on a course of mindfulness. You can be confident that if you commit yourself to the practices, you will be sure to benefit. The evidence of the effectiveness of mindfulness is now well established through all the research that has and is taking place.

However, there are some definite challenges to learning to be mindful and it helps to be prepared for them.

Courage and compassion

Mindfulness is NOT about feeling relaxed and calm – however appealing that may sound. It involves us in developing the capacity to be attentive and aware of present moment experience. Some aspects of this, as we become steadier, involve us in becoming more aware of what challenges us.

Our basic instinct is to pull away from what we dislike or find difficult. Although this is natural, the way we do this can add to our struggles. Instead, with practice, we discover that mindfulness offers us a way of relating more gently to experience by coming alongside our difficulties with kindness – befriending them rather than fighting or running away from them. This might call for a measure of courage at times.

Establishing a mindfulness practice

In order to develop mindfulness into a significant personal resource, we first have to establish the ground of the practice. This requires time, practice and effort. We have not even started yet and 'practice' has already been mentioned many times!

As with any approach that has the potential to offer a lot, it would be dishonest to imply that the benefits of mindfulness are easily gained. The reality for most of us is that it needs sustained effort and committed practice.

However, we all engage with things differently – at different times. What may be right for one person at one time may be unwise for another. There are no prescriptions. It is for you to decide. You have every choice from following the approach methodically, to dipping in and out, and to everything in between. Most of us come to mindfulness practice incrementally. Seeds get sown and germinate at different times – and some never 'take' at all.

How will you decide on your level of engagement?

Throughout the chapters, you are encouraged to follow a number of practices, preferably daily. As has been described, there is one longer core practice and two short practices in each chapter. This may seem like a lot. It would not help to keep reminding you of your choice not to do this – so the approach is to encourage you throughout. In the next chapter, we look at cultivating your intention to support you with this. For now – reflecting on the following question:

What will help me to commit to following the practices?

Embarking on establishing a mindfulness practice is a bit like going for a walk in the country. Some of it is lovely. We want to linger and enjoy it. Some places feel familiar, and link us to where we have been before. Other parts feel like hard work, and even boring and monotonous. Can you approach it all with openness and curiosity – not anticipating difficulties, nor expecting results? Just seeing what is here for now. You can feel justifiably happy at the end of each practice having completed what you intended.

Committing to a practice is not a steady process. As with most new habits – it tends to be a business of starting, lapsing, coming back and beginning again – over and over. Most of us find it to be so.

We look at this at different points, but as you start out now, remembering what has drawn you to mindfulness and resolve to be ready to come back and begin again as many times as you need to. In my experience people with cancer do well with mindfulness. Most are highly motivated to find the tools that will help them manage anxiety and troublesome states of mind, so that they no longer seem to define them. As a result, people with cancer tend to be committed to their practice and benefit in many ways.

Embarking on your own via a book is quite challenging. Attending a course and learning alongside others helps us to keep going, week-by-week. However, there are advantages here in being able to take your time and adapting things to suit you. Some of you may be able to use this book alongside an eight–week course, currently or recently.

And finally

Those involved in writing and producing this book have done their best to make it as easy to follow as possible. However, any mistakes within these pages are entirely mine, as author. I have tried to find a balance between optimism and realism. It is sometimes a fine line to negotiate and there may be places where I have not managed it. I hope these do not hinder your learning.

Anything you gain from this approach will be due to your commitment and good heart. I hope that you get much benefit and that your life is enriched with mindfulness and kindness.

Notes

1 Rumi, J.B. (1999) By kind permission of Penguin Books.
2 Rilke, R.M. (1934)
3 See mindfulness and cancer research headlines in Appendix 1.
4 Kabat-Zinn, J. (1990, 2013)
5 Segal, Z.V., Williams, J.M.G., & Teasdale, J.D. (2013)
6 Bartley, T. (2012)
7 See the Rilke quotation at the start of the chapter.
8 The website www.thoughtonathread.co.uk will give you more information about how the threads first came to be used through a connection with a South African community based project called Woza Moya, which supports people affected by HIV & Aids.

Chapter 1

Intention

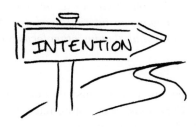

May what I do flow from me like a river,
no forcing and no holding back,
the way it is with children.

Then in these swelling and ebbing currents,
these deepening tides moving out, returning,
I will sing you as no one ever has,
streaming through widening channels
into the open sea.

Rainer Maria Rilke[1]

This poem might be speaking about learning to be mindful in the context of cancer. A small river is always flowing and changing. Sometimes it is bright and dancing, sometimes agitated and busy, and sometimes depleted and low. Yet, streams and rivers can fascinate in their movement, flow, and inevitable journey to the sea. Do you have a river near you? Could you go and watch it with this idea of flow and change in mind?

Rilke is speaking of his intention, 'May what I do flow from me like a river'. I think he is inviting the possibility of being entirely how he is, moment by moment – inspired by the river that has no way of being anything else. We so often try to be braver and better. Is it possible to be the river that you are?

Mindfulness: A Kindly Approach to Being with Cancer, First Edition. Trish Bartley.
© 2017 John Wiley & Sons, Ltd. Published 2017 by John Wiley & Sons, Ltd.
Companion Website: www.wiley.com/go/bartley/mindfulness

Intention

The intentions we set ourselves remind us of what is important. It is like having an internal compass. When we form the intention to be more mindful, that intention focuses and shapes our choices and actions.

Myla and Jon Kabat-Zinn[2]

Intention is the first of our four movements, underpinning all the others. Consciously cultivating intention may not be a familiar process – but if we identify and stay connected with what matters to us, it will support us well. Maybe, we can then use our time to make space to enjoy what is precious. We can choose to stop delaying living – and allow an experience of illness to motivate choices of wellness. What might that mean to you? There may be lots of reasons why this may not seem possible, but let us see what unfolds from the process of cultivating mindful intention.

We consider this in a number of ways that are practical, reflective and practice-based. Later, we follow a Body Scan, and introduce two short practices. At the end of this chapter, we look at the implications of being diagnosed with cancer, and learn a 'first aid' mindfulness practice.

Preparing the ground[3]

Cultivating intention is the first step in bringing mindfulness into your life. It links you to your vision for what you hope mindfulness may offer.

We might bring to mind some intentions made in the past that started well, but did not last. Like New Year's Resolutions, they often focus on giving something up, rather than putting something in place. The motivation behind them is what seems to count. Cultivating an 'ought to' intention is likely to become irritating and guilt inducing. At the other extreme, we might be tempted to frame our intention in meaningful significance that is writ large! This can prove exhausting to sustain.

Our world tends to motivate us towards hard work and constant busyness. We end up driven to get more and more done. When someone becomes ill, their productivity is inevitably diminished and this can feel very difficult, for the universe tends to define us by what we do – as we do ourselves.

Instead can we look at intentions that support a simpler and kinder way of being? Can we find ways of fostering a commitment to enjoy and appreciate all that we love in our lives? Can we put meaning into the detail of 'living' rather than the 'doing' of it? This is what mindfulness has to offer us.

Intention has a vital role in 'co-opting' your mind to come onboard as an ally and a friend.

When mindfulness is harnessed with conscious intention, we can align to those choices that support well-being and offer skilful responses to difficulty.

Developing a new skill takes practice. Starting mindfulness is a bit like learning to play a musical instrument. It takes time before you can make a decent sound – but with a commitment to practice regularly, it starts to feel more natural.

Every action involves some form of intention. It might be vague – an almost *mindless* or unconscious intention – such as when we stand up to make a hot drink, or walk upstairs to fetch something and then forget half way up what we wanted!

At the other end of the scale, there are *overarching* intentions that are formed to support what is wholesome – and what we hold dear. These then become *specific* when translated into everyday actions. They guide the choices we make.

Jennifer was going to be 40 and had finished treatment for breast cancer two years before. She decided to enter her first ever mini triathlon to prove to herself that she was now well and not yet 'over the hill' (her **overarching intention**). She made some **specific intentions** to train regularly in all three activities. She didn't do as much as she planned, but she was thrilled to be able to complete the course.

Clarifying Your Intention

We look now at cultivating a personal overarching intention. There are three steps to follow, which you will be guided through. This may seem a bit mechanical for something that connects you with what you hold dear, so you might reflect on some of this on a walk, while listening to some lovely music, or in conversation with a friend.

It will help to record your reflections and the answers to your questions, in your notebook if you like – so that you can refer back to them later.

- The **first step** focuses on how you are now and what has drawn you to mindfulness.
- The **second step** invites you to explore your personal vision, values and aspirations. These are the things in your life that you care most about.
- Finally, **in the third step**, you will be guided through an intention practice. This will help you identify your overarching intentions in the light of the previous two steps.

Following this process may make all the difference to what you get from the approach in this book.

The first step

What draws you to mindfulness?
Recording how things are now gives you a reference point for the future.

Current levels of stress
What impact has cancer diagnosis and treatment had on you?

- How stressed have you felt over the last few weeks? Is this generally more or less than over the last few months?
- Give yourself a score from 1–10 (10 is highest stress – 1 is lowest) relating to how you are <u>now</u>.
- What are the key signs of stress currently (sleeping? eating? physical symptoms? mood? energy? emotions? troubling thoughts?)? Be as detailed as you can, recording what gives you most trouble and how.
- Record today's date alongside these answers.

Specific hopes

EITHER

You encountered mindfulness before you were diagnosed and may have (or have had) an existing practice.
OR
You are new to mindfulness, but have heard or read about it, and want to know more.

What do you hope that the mindfulness approach in this book will offer you? Be as specific as you can.

Mindfulness and cancer

Knowing how mindfulness has benefited others can help you to develop trust in this approach – even though everyone gets something different.

There are two perspectives on offer to you. Having taught mindfulness to many people with cancer, in 8 week courses and also one-to-one, I often notice that those who commit to the practices as fully as they can, positively benefit from the process. It is never possible to predict the shape and form of this, but as you will read, some people's experience of life is greatly changed for the better after learning mindfulness. My colleagues see similar outcomes with people with cancer. Learning to live more mindfully enables people to develop and use tools that help them manage their challenging feelings. As a result, they feel more content.

Another perspective can be drawn from the research. Evidence of the benefits of mindfulness for people with cancer is established and growing. Linda Carlson and her team in Canada have extensively researched this over many years.[4] Mindfulness-based approaches have been found to be effective for people with cancer across a range of outcomes, including stress symptoms, mood, fatigue, quality of life, and sleep symptoms. Overall levels of anxiety and depression were found to reduce and overall levels of well-being were found to increase. Researchers have much more to discover, but there are some early findings that suggest some physical benefits from practicing mindfulness that relate to biomarkers, which may link with the impact of stress on the immune system.

The second step

Personal vision, values and aspirations

We start by asking a key question and inviting you to reflect on it.

What really matters to me?

Time rushes by and another year passes. We seem to experience chunks of life almost as if half asleep – existing much of the time in automatic mode.

Sometimes, getting cancer can illuminate this. Mindfulness helps people with cancer find more meaning and purpose in their lives – often through a greater sense of interconnectedness with others. It is vital that we relate to the things that matter most to us. If we fail to do this, they will pass us by. We will not realize their significance or make choices that are aligned to them.

Jack Kornfield voices this in his book *A Path with Heart*:

In the stress and complexity of our lives, we may forget our deepest intentions. But when people come to the end of their life and look back, the questions they most often ask are not usually, 'How much is in my bank account?'… or 'What did I build?' or the like. ……The questions such a person asks are very simple: 'Did I love well?' Did I live fully?[5]

Dr. Atul Gawande, surgeon and author, makes a similar point in a different context, as he challenges medicine and his medical colleagues:

We've been wrong about what our job is in medicine. We think our job is to ensure health and survival. But really it is larger than that. It is to enable well-being. And well-being is about the reasons one wishes to be alive.[6]

What really matters to me?

Sitting and breathing with this question – and maybe walking with it. Encouraging you to pause and take your time to shape your answer to this.

Miriam had been treated for cancer for several years and found sadly that her life now felt much reduced. However, when she thought about what really mattered to her, she found so much. 'I had to put things in groups, or my list would have been too long to remember', she told me. 'Beauty really matters, and nature, and the walnut tree in the garden that looks like a Bedouin tent – and of course my family, especially my children – and when I thought about it, I realized how important laughter is to me, especially with my five special friends. We share such a sense of the ridiculous!' she finished, sounding happy and animated.

When you have reflected and written as much as you want, move on to step three.

The third step

Now is the time to follow the intentions practice from the website. After this you will be invited to write a letter to yourself.

The words below are simply for guidance. They are very similar to those on the website recording.

 An intentions practice

Settling into a comfortable position ... Imagining that you are standing or sitting beside a body of water – a lake, or a stream or the ocean itself. The water beside you is very clear and you can see all the way down to the bottom. Choosing an imaginary pebble, holding it in your hand, and then tossing it gently into the water – watching it sink very, very, slowly (much more slowly than it actually would). Asking yourself ...

- *'What really matters to me?'*
- *'What do I most wish for myself?'*
- *'What is my intention in relation to mindfulness and this book?'*

Not being concerned if answers don't come, just continuing to ask gently, opening to the possibility of something emerging from within you – maybe some thoughts, maybe some feelings – perhaps some inner wisdom. Keep asking as you imagine that you see the pebble gently sink through the water. Eventually the pebble comes to rest ...

Intentions letter

EITHER

- Write yourself a kindly letter, describing the intentions that emerged for you during the practice.
  OR
- If your best friend was talking to you about mindfulness and what this book might offer you, what wise advice and gentle encouragement might s/he offer?

Intentions Letter

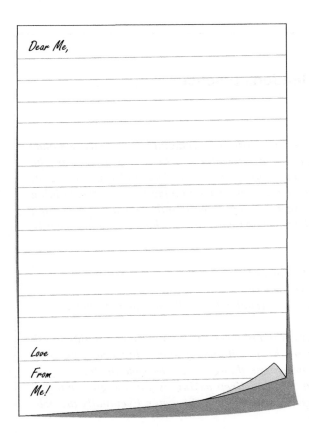

Dear Me,

Love
From
Me!

Here are three examples of intentions letters. They were all written at the start of mindfulness journeys – and much later, the authors of the letters kindly offered to share them for this book.

Kate was caring for her husband who had incurable cancer. Both his daughters also had cancer. She had the tendency to get angry when she was under pressure. Her intentions letter speaks of this:

> I hope I grow in wisdom. I hope I find a way to walk beside this family with love and kindness. I hope I find ways to cool the heat of my rage. I hope I find the strength to live alone without him and have no regrets for the way we share this time.

June had recently finished treatment for breast cancer when she started her course. A devoted grandmother, she was surrounded by a busy extended family, yet she often felt alone with her fears:

> I hope mindfulness will give me the courage to be stronger in moments of despair. I want to live life to the full without being overwhelmed by the fears and worries that surround the thoughts of cancer and what is happening inside my body. I will give this course my total commitment to that end.

George, an elderly man with terminal cancer, was in a very anxious place when he started mindfulness. His letter speaks of the courage he wants to cultivate and of what and who matters most to him:

> I've embarked on this to learn to be braver in the face of my illness. I want to be able to attain some stillness (Be still my soul!) and be thankful for all life has given me over the years. I want especially not to burden my family with destructive self-pity and to show them how much I love them and appreciate their love of me. Can I learn to love myself despite everything?

Specific intentions

Later, we will learn to translate the overarching intentions that you write about in your letter, into specific commitments. By linking regularly with intention, we let what matters to us underpin our actions and practices. We will learn to pause regularly, as this gives us time to remember.

There might be some special contexts or moments that need particular intentions – such as when you go to clinic or are waiting to receive results. You will learn some practices that support waiting and treatment times, later in the book.

For now, having written your letter and reflected on each of the steps, you have made a good start. You have laid down some significant foundations that will hold and support you as you bring mindfulness into your life.

Three skilful intentions

There are three powerful partners in cultivating mindfulness: *kindness, compassion* and *being with.*

Kindness

Mindfulness practice is infused with a quality of **kindness**. This is very different to the attitude of mind that habitually judges and takes things personally. When we bring a friendly attention to what is happening, this spills over into how we are with others, and how we experience our world.

Sheila found it helped her to connect with kindness when she brought to mind how she was with her children, and how her mother was with her. This helped her develop kindness towards herself. It was not an easy process for her, but she got more and more glimpses of it as she practiced.

Compassion

Is a kindly way of meeting pain and suffering. Instead of closing down and tightening against it, we learn to gently open to what is there – whether it is emotional distress, or physical pain, in us or in others. We learn that it is not so much *my* pain, but *the* pain that anyone in this situation might feel. Compassion is sometimes called the 'trembling of the heart'. It enables us to take the action that is needed, inspired by a wish to ease suffering.

Jane got to know many of the others who regularly had chemo with her. She cared about them and what happened to them. Later in the mindfulness course, she brought them to mind and how it had been. 'I really feel for everyone who has to go through chemo as we did', she said, 'It helped me so much to have others there, experiencing the same as me. Feeling for them, I could somehow be more patient and caring with myself.'

Being with

Helps us to cultivate a wiser and less reactive way of being. By coming back to the resonance of sensations in the body, we notice when troublesome thoughts and emotions arise. Instead of getting stuck in deepening loops of negativity, we can acknowledge the struggle and hold it gently in the body. We are cultivating the possibility of freeing the mind in the moment, from the stuck places that state, 'I am (or it is) always like this' – and suggesting that in the midst of it all, we can be with it in awareness, kindness and compassion.

Everything new needs to be held, needs a place into which it can be born.[7]

Concluding

Cultivating and clarifying intentions for living mindfully is time well spent, however long this takes you. If you have not reflected on your intentions yet, it is worth going back, before moving on to the next section, where we learn to bring mindfulness into the context of living with cancer.

My Late Night Visitor

I sit propped up in my bed
comfortable, relaxed.
Pen in hand I am trying to write a poem.

"Can I get into your bed?"
No pause for my possible reply
Teddy under one arm, pillow under the other
She climbs across me to the other side of the bed.
She arranges her pillow to her satisfaction,
Settles herself with teddy and goes straight to sleep.
We have not spoken a word.

I put down my pen and give in to the moment.
I watch her sleep, I count her breaths.
Have those freckles always been there across her nose?
Her face is beautiful and the more I examine it
The less I seem to know it.
Did my mother gaze like this at me when I was five?
Will my daughter in turn gaze at her daughter when she is five?
I feel a sense of my place in the grand scheme of things
It feels right, it feels good.

She opens her eyes and gives me a steady look.
With a sleepy half smile she turns over and faces the wall.
I pick up my pen.

Liz

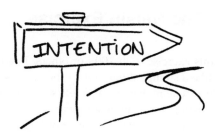

The Practice of Mindfulness

Overview

We begin with a traditional introduction to mindfulness – and then go on to encounter one of the key practices, which become part of your daily menu for the next weeks. We also explore ways of approaching home practice – so that your intentions are put to good use in everyday routines.

Two groups of people travel with you throughout this book. There are those who have been on similar journeys themselves, and know the lie of the land. They share some practice stories with you.

The others are your fellow travellers, reading as you read, and practicing as you practice. Together, you form a community of mindfulness practitioners with cancer. You can wish them well, now at the start and at any other time along the way – just as you can be sure that they wish you well. You may never see their faces, but as time passes and your understanding and practice deepens, you will know that they too lie awake worrying just like you; and they too feel the sun on their backs and experience the joy of being alive, just like you. We are so different in so many ways, yet we share so much in the landscape of what we find distressing and what gives us joy. Strangely, when we connect with this, it helps us not to feel so alone.

The Raisin Exercise

I first experienced this exercise with 100s of others, in a huge hall in central London. It seemed like a strange thing to do, especially with so many people. I was in the middle of chemotherapy and felt self-conscious with my head scarf. Yet it was interesting to reflect on afterwards.

My voice will guide you from the website recording. I will be following the practice myself as I lead it for you. This is your first taste of mindfulness. You are joining many thousands of others who have been introduced to mindfulness in just the same way. You may have experienced this exercise before. Even if you have, it is helpful to do it again. See if you can come fresh to the raisin, as if you have no idea what it is, and no expectations of what we will be doing ...

Have a raisin ready when you follow this practice.

The Raisin Exercise

Your first taste of mindfulness! – Imagine that you have dropped in from Mars and have no idea what this little object is in the hand! Feel it in the palm ... ... have a good look at it (taking your time and focusing in on all the detail that you can see); ... ... bring it up to the nose and smell it slowly; ... ... feel the touch of it in your fingers (maybe closing your eyes to focus in on the texture); ... ... and finally and very slowly, place it in the mouth. Chewing deliberately and slowly one chew at a time, ... noticing the taste, the texture, the experience of swallowing, ...

We approach things 'as if for the first time' by bringing a fresh awake curiosity to the experience of the little raisin. Some of you may enjoy the strange oddness of it. Others of you may be bored and become restless with the slowness of it. Whatever you feel, see if you can simply explore your experience of the raisin, and this exercise, using the following questions – almost as if to gently get some juice out of the little thing.

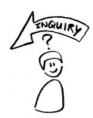

Reflective inquiry

- What was happening for you as you went through the different parts of the raisin exercise?
- What did you notice – in detail – about the raisin?
- How was it to experience a raisin in this way?

Try the raisin exercise with younger family members, you may learn from their 'beginners mind'. I did this with my 7-year-old granddaughter. She noticed the shapes on the surface of the raisin and liked the way they reflected light – and she laughed, delighted at the tiny sound the raisin made when she squished it near her ear. She later announced in a family meal that she would like to listen to her vegetables rather than eat them!

A definition of mindfulness

Jon Kabat-Zinn defines mindfulness as 'the awareness that emerges when we:

pay attention
on purpose
in the present moment
without judgment
in the service of greater self-understanding, wisdom and well-being.'[8]

Spending a little time now reflecting on the raisin exercise in the context of this definition.

- What was the particular way that you paid attention?
- What do the other aspects of the definition mean to you – on purpose; in the present moment and without judgement?

When I lead this with a group of people with cancer, participants often comment on the way we slowed down. They describe what they noticed with each sense, one at a time. Some people associate the smell of the raisin with Christmas, or the kitchen they remember as children. Others realize how often they taste things without really tasting them at all. Some of them describe how much they did NOT want to taste the raisin. We learn that taking time to be present to the taste, and smell, and look of something changes the experience. We notice more. It is so different to chucking a handful of raisins in the mouth and swallowing them after a very few chews. Wanting a 'hit' of sweetness, the mouthful passes almost unnoticed in a second.

Stephen was unsure about the whole mindfulness enterprize, but his wife had persuaded him to give it a go and join a course. 'It came as a bit of a shock on that first day when we were given that raisin. I was sceptical – but then I was intrigued. It seemed such a trivial thing to do, but it obviously had quite enormous resonance, once you grasped the fact that eating the raisin is a metaphor for all sorts of things. After that, I began to look at it all with more interest.

Eating mindfully at home

In the weeks to come, see if you can bring the same curious fresh attention to the taste of your food from time to time. Pausing at some point to look at, smell, and taste one mouthful. What do you notice? There is no right way to do this, nor do you need to be enjoying the food – you are simply aware of tasting in that very moment. You are waking up to the process of eating, instead of automatically chewing and swallowing, without tasting much at all.

Margret attended a mindfulness course in a nearby community hall. She was known in the neighbourhood to love her cups of tea. She might have twenty or more a day and had done for years. After tasting the raisin in the first class, she returned the next week in some consternation. She had mindfully drunk a cup of tea – and discovered that she did not like the taste!

Short Practices

The Pause

This is a key practice that helps us to reconnect with our present moment experience. It is simplicity itself, yet it holds an important key – for the more we practice the Pause, the more we build the 'muscle' that enables us to remember to interrupt the automatic and come back to what is happening *here and now*.

The Pause

Begin by stopping what you are doing – and asking yourself one of the following questions:

- *What is going on for me right now?*
  or
- *How am I feeling right now?*

Keep this very simple. You might want to adapt the question to make it your own. You are feeling into *a sense of what is happening in this moment – not so much* thinking about *it.*

Practicing the Pause

Practicing this several times a day over the next two or more weeks helps you to develop the habit of interrupting the automatic way we live so much of our lives – pausing and coming back.

- You might choose to practice the Pause every time you do a specific task such as: at the start of meals; when you open email; in the middle of washing up; as you go outside.
  or
- You might choose to practice a Pause whenever you notice you are feeling: speedy; anxious; stressed; irritable; or upset.

Feet on the Floor

This is your second key short practice in this chapter. Like the Pause it is straightforward – deceptively so. It appears to be something of nothing – yet many people find that bringing attention to the sensations of feet on the floor, whether sitting or standing, offers them a reliable anchor to come back to, over and over. It forms the basis of the beginning of many subsequent short practices.

Feet on the Floor

Feeling the contact of your feet on the ground … … just placing your attention down onto the soles of your feet and noticing whatever is there. Exploring the detailed sensations in your toes, (are they all in contact with your shoes or the floor or do some have more contact than others?) … … … the balls of the feet (what is the shape of that contact?), and the heels (what is the quality of the contact? – how does it feel?). Perhaps feeling the texture of the shoes surrounding the feet … … perhaps moving to the feel of the solid of the floor beneath you. Noticing the weight of you going down, through your legs onto your feet, on the floor. Just being curious about all of this – and keep bringing the mind back to the sensations of contact with the floor.

Practice this for a few moments – regularly several times a day – maybe linking it to a daily activity (such as getting out of bed, or boiling the kettle, or waiting in a queue, or finishing a meal).

You can do this at any time, wherever you are; sitting, standing, walking, and lying down. If you are walking – you simply notice the moment the foot comes down onto the ground. If you wake in the night, or have trouble getting to sleep, you can practice this by bringing attention to the contact of your body with the mattress or the bedding; noticing all the different sensations of contact between your body and the bed.

The key is to remember to do it. There is no need to do it for long periods – a few seconds at a time is fine. This is one of the building blocks that form your 'cancer' practices later on – so cultivating your intention to practice is important to ensure it becomes an established part of your mindfulness repertoire, whenever you need it. Following this several times a day for at least two weeks will help you integrate it into your life. Bringing specific intention to do this at the start is very helpful and then being curious about the experience of doing it.

- When do you plan to practice Feet on the Floor?
- What activity will you attach it to?
- How will you remember?

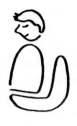

Core Practice

The Body Scan

This is your first core practice. It lasts for about 30 minutes. You can use the script below to guide you – but it is better to download the guided Body Scan from the website and follow it. It has been recorded specifically for you to use with this book. Find a way of doing it regularly in a place that is comfortable for you.

Posture
You can follow this practice lying down, on the floor, on a bed, or on a couch. Alternatively, it may prefer to sit in a comfortable chair, with your head and legs supported. You may want a rug or blanket over you, and pillows to support your head, and under your knees. The idea is for you to be comfortable, warm and well supported, and also awake and alert.

Body Scan Practice

'Settling into the sensations of contact of your body with the floor, or bed, or chair as you briefly scan through the body from the feet up to the head ... ... adjusting any part of you that wants to move to a more comfortable position ... ... maybe your head and neck – or your back ... ... checking to see what might be needed...... and then becoming aware of the detailed qualities of contact between your body and what you are lying on ... ...

When you are ready, moving attention deliberately to the breath breathing deep in the body, perhaps placing your hands on the belly to guide you ... and simply resting awareness on the movement of the belly under the hands, as the breath comes in and goes out ... not changing it in any way, letting it breathe exactly as it does, without trying to control it in any way ... ...

We are now going to practice The Body Scan.

As we begin, connect with your intention for this practice. Feel this within you, letting your intention guide you throughout the practice. Remembering there is no specific goal to attain. The invitation is simply to follow as best you can, bringing your attention to the sensations in the different parts of your body and exploring them as I guide you through the practice. Remembering that it is fine if you find that you do not want to do something that I invite you to do, but always choosing and doing what is best for you. At any time, you may choose to ignore my practice and come back to the breath, breathing deep in the belly, as you are aware of it now ... ...

Now, when you are ready, moving your attention from the belly all the way down to the left foot and then out to the toes of the left foot ... ... noticing any sensations in the big toe – perhaps contact with the sock or stocking, maybe warmth or coolness, throbbing or tickling, a sense of the shape of the toe, maybe teasing out sensations of toe nail or pad of the toe .... (then moving through the different toes, and parts of toes and foot – inviting noticing of sensations, and texture, heat, hardness and softness, contact, inside and outside, and so on ...) ...

If you find as we do this, that you notice that some areas don't have much sensation, then see if you can explore what 'not much sensation' feels like ... ... remembering we are just practicing being aware and whatever you notice is fine ... ... we are not trying to change any part of your experience, just practicing being aware of how it is.

When you are ready, turning to the breath again, and imagine that you can breathe in a different way – bringing the breath all the way down the left side of the body, through the left leg, into the left foot and the left toes, as you are if breathing into the foot and then breathing out from the foot, up through the body and out through the nose. It is as if we are using the breath as a vehicle for our awareness ... ... On the next out breath, letting go of this focus on the breath and the left foot, and moving up through the ankle to the left lower leg ... ... (repeating this process through all the different sections of the body – sometimes widening the beam of attention to take in the whole of a limb or the whole of the trunk of the body ...) ...

If at any point you notice that your mind has wandered off into thinking, or you have been distracted by something such as a sound, or drawn to some other part of the body, simply noticing where the mind has got to, and gently and kindly bringing your focus back to wherever we have got to in the body ... ... If at any point, we come to an area that holds pain, or discomfort or difficult feelings for you, seeing if it is possible to pause ... ... perhaps bringing the breath gently down into and around the area, and breathing into it and breathing out from it with kindness and sensitivity ... ... not trying to change it, but simply to offer this area some kindly attention ... ... noticing if the mind moves into thoughts about it, and if it does, seeing if you can simply come back to the sensations in the body, wherever you are choosing to focus ... ...

As we come to the end of this practice, expanding the attention into a sense of the body as a whole lying here ... ... and coming to the breath, breathing into and out from the whole of the body ... ... Now, if you would like to, gently turning towards any part of your body that has experienced treatment or injury – or feels tender or painful at the moment. Inviting you to bring gentleness and kindness to this part – breathing into it gently, if this feels ok, and opening to any sensations that are present there, and holding them gently in awareness ... ... now, when you are ready, coming back to a sense of the whole of the body again, bringing any awareness of tenderness into a sense of the whole body. And when you are ready, taking your time to open your eyes and perhaps moving any parts of the body that would like to move. Getting up (if you choose) and deciding what you will do next.

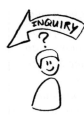

Reflective inquiry

- What was happening for you as you went through the different parts of the Body Scan?
- What did you notice, in general and more specifically?
- How was it to experience your body in this way?

You are invited to reflect like this on all the practices that you follow, especially the guided core practices. You can develop and adapt your own questions. It helps to spend a few moments at the end of each practice, pausing and noticing what you experienced. You can use your notebook or reflect internally. There is often a temptation to get to the end and move straight back into activity and busyness. See if you can take your time, bringing mindful awareness back with you into whatever comes next.

Practicing the Body Scan

You are encouraged to practice the Body Scan at least ten times before you move on to the next chapter. Ideally, you might practice it every day – but some days will be easier than others, so we are aiming for ten times over a fortnight – or twenty Body Scans over a month.

Decide when might be the best time to suit your day and choose a place where you are unlikely to be disturbed. Let your family know that you will be doing this most days – and ask for their support in not interrupting you. Make a choice not to take your phone with you – and then you can dedicate this time to you and your well-being. Morning may be a better time than evening as this offers a better chance of staying awake – but explore what works best for you. In the next chapter, we will learn more about the Body Scan. For now, it is best to experience it in your own way.

Intention

See if you can bring your intention into your plans to practice the Body Scan, the Pause and Feet on the Floor. By translating your overarching intention (what really matters to me?) into everyday commitments, little by little, and day by day, you are supporting the way you want to live. You are aligning your choices to supporting the life you want. Each recorded practice starts with intention. You might even start each day by connecting with your practice intention for that day.

The Experience of Cancer

In the final section of each chapter, we focus on different aspects in the experience of cancer. These follow a chronological order, although this will not necessarily align with your experience. In this section, we touch on the impact of diagnosis and learn a 'first aid' mindfulness practice. There are also descriptions of approaches and activities that others have found helpful.

Diagnosis

Getting a diagnosis of cancer is deeply shocking. Medicine and science have made great advances in the research and treatment of cancer – yet when one of us, or someone we care about, is given a cancer diagnosis, we feel shocked and distressed. We immediately fear the worst.

Sandra (50) was living on her own and just back from working overseas as a teacher. She attended the clinic after finding a small lump in her left breast. She remembers feeling incredibly thirsty straight after being told it was cancer. The nurse went to get her some water, but came back with the tiniest of cups and had to go back again and again to get more. 'I felt very upset and shaky. I remember the doctor giving me endless information and thinking to myself, "How can he possibly imagine I can take all of this in?" Yet somewhere inside, I had noticed that he had mentioned four possible treatments, and I vowed there and then that I wouldn't agree to having them all – and I didn't.'

Why me? Why now?

Getting a cancer diagnosis challenges the assumption that we have control over our lives. When tragedy strikes, we invariably hunt for a cause, desperately trying to wrestle back some sense of certainty. We look at who or what is at fault. We blame ourselves. 'If I had gone to the doctor earlier, this might not have happened.' 'I must have done something to deserve this.'

Rationally, it is important to acknowledge that cancer describes a wide range of illnesses with multiple causes, some of which are not yet well understood. Even if we made unwise choices in the past, most of the causes and conditions for getting cancer are beyond our control. Reflecting on this, can you untangle yourself from the additional suffering of self-blame?

The psychological impact

The discovery of life threatening illness and the need for arduous treatments has a strong physical and emotional impact. If at the same time, you are told that your illness is incurable, many people feel they are left without hope. For a time, they may feel quite unable to carry on. It is not surprising that anxiety or depression is significant in people recently diagnosed with cancer,[9] whatever their prognosis. Overall, it is considered that at least 25–30% of people with cancer suffer from cancer-related psychological disorders.[9]

A cancer diagnosis often comes at the end of a period of waiting and worrying. I know someone who put an oncology appointment letter right at the back of a cupboard, and told no-one about it until a few days before she was due at the hospital. The worst possible outcome may have been imagined many times – and yet it is still a considerable shock when it comes.

Mary (65) was soon to be a grandmother when she was diagnosed with ovarian cancer. She remembers sitting in a large hospital clinic with her partner, waiting to see the doctor to get her test results. She realized that some people, sitting alongside her, would be told they had cancer that day. 'Everyone looked so pale and scared. I remember wishing the best for all those who were going to be diagnosed that day – never thinking I would be one. I really thought I was ok – and that we were just being careful and getting things checked out. I was later told that there were eight of us that afternoon.'

Waiting

More waiting follows the actual diagnosis – waiting for test results; waiting to see what treatments are recommended; waiting to be referred to another specialty; waiting to hear about a research trial; waiting, waiting. These periods are hard – involving feelings of helplessness and intense anxiety. We tend to move from one extreme to another – from optimism to despair – from feeling it is manageable, to feeling it is impossible to endure.

Until relatively recently, patients were shielded from their diagnosis, and not even told they had cancer. Overprotective attitudes in medical practice are relatively rare now in most societies. We are usually told about the implications of the diagnosis and what treatment is likely to be needed. Whilst this is a great improvement on what used to happen, the traumatic impact of being given a diagnosis is often not fully recognized by medical practitioners.

It is quite normal to react initially to diagnosis with shock and disbelief. Many people describe feelings of numbness and unreality, often accompanied by racing thoughts and a sense of disconnection from the people and events around them. There are however a wide range of reactions to diagnosis. Some people appear not to react much at all.

> Patrik (44), originally from Norway had moved to the UK 10 years before, to work in the health service. He had a young family. He cannot remember much about his diagnosis of bladder cancer. 'I was on my own for the appointment, I remember that. I had not told Elizabeth anything about it. It was certainly a surprise, but I am a pretty optimistic person and felt quite confident about my prognosis. I just wanted to hear about the treatment options, and get on with it as soon as possible.'

After some of the shock has worn off, anger, anxiety and depression may follow. Slowly most people adjust in time to the implications of a cancer diagnosis, although longer-term psychological difficulties can persist even after treatment has finished.

Some likely reactions

Not surprisingly, many people experience feelings of numbness and shock.

> John could hardly hear what the doctor was saying. It was as if he was being talked to from a long, long distance away.

Others may feel quite overwhelmed and have catastrophic thoughts.

> Debbie spent hours and hours on the Internet, reading about her type of cancer. She was convinced that she would die and became increasingly distressed.

Others appear to take the news in their stride.

> Rebecca went straight back to work and carried on as if nothing had happened. But she woke up several nights in a row sobbing in her sleep. 'I was so surprised when I got up the following morning. I thought I had been coping so well', she told me.

Sometimes intrusive memories of the diagnosis break through at odd times of the day and night.

> Ellen hated going back to the clinic where she had received news of her diagnosis. She had vivid memories of the room, the nurse, the doctor and a particular notice on the wall about fire drill. She would find herself reliving it, remembering it in detail, especially at night.

We are all different. Each of us reacts in our own way. There is no better or worse way to react than any other, although it may not always feel like that. We tend to assume that people who are stoical and do not obviously get upset may be managing 'the best', but that is not necessarily borne out. Our reactions depend very much on our own style of coping, and a multitude of different circumstances, present and past. It is all too easy to judge ourselves for the way we feel.

Reflecting on your own diagnosis

Maybe some of these stories resonate with how it was for you – maybe not. If you feel it might be helpful to reflect a bit on your own diagnosis and how you felt at the time, you might want to do this internally or perhaps in your notebook.

On the other hand, if it all seems too close and too difficult, there is no need to push yourself into this. Instead, you can go to the short practice at the end of this section and see what it offers you.

The following questions might be a starting point for your reflection, if you choose to do it:

- What or who was helpful for you at the diagnosis?
- Do you remember your first reactions? Were you mostly aware of your feelings and emotions, or your thoughts, or the sensations in your body? Or was your attention focused outward on what was going around you?
- Looking back on that time, how do you feel towards yourself now?
- If you were talking to someone who had just been told they had cancer – what might you say to them?

The period between diagnosis and the start of treatment can be tough. It always involves periods of waiting – for results, for news, for appointments, for tests. There is so much uncertainty. It is new territory for most of us and we have so much to learn about how the system works and what to expect.

- What could you suggest to others going through a similar time that you found helpful?

Here are a few ideas from various people I have asked.

Eating in the early days after diagnosis

> Jerry: 'I found it very hard to face food. My appetite vanished. It was as if my system had shut down – but I could manage soup. It had to be quite bland, especially to begin with – and warm and smooth. But it felt comforting and easy to digest.'[10]

Walking

> Matt: 'When I did the mindfulness course the year before, I really liked the mindful walking. So when I got diagnosed, I decided to walk a bit every day. My mind was endlessly slipping into *"what if?"* or *"what have I done to deserve this?"* Walking was the only way I could get any peace. It didn't always work – but if I concentrated on the air on my face, or my feet touching the ground – I felt more calm somehow, sometimes anyway.'

Writing

> Jenny poured her experience into her journal. She wrote down all her feelings about what had happened. As the weeks passed, she started collecting things to put in the pages. Some leaves from a walk – a sketch of the café table where she met a friend – a newspaper cutting – a message from her daughter. She used a big rubber band to hold it together.

Music

> Mary was a member of the local choir and loved music. After she was diagnosed, she would find a quiet space in the day and choose some music that spoke of how she was feeling or what she felt she needed. Sometimes, it would be a sad piece – sometimes something that was slow and soothing. She let the sounds flow into her, as if comforting her sad, frightened heart.

Gardening

> David spent many hours in the garden after he got his news. He could lose himself tending the plants and trees – and forget things for a moment or two. It helped him to stay active. He often wondered how he would cope without the garden to work in.

A 'First Aid' Practice

 The time following diagnosis is often marked by intense anxiety and uncertainty. Things change very quickly from how life had been before the diagnosis. There may also be a sense of dislocation at home, with heightened feelings – and the phone constantly ringing and people visiting. Or maybe it is the opposite – with silence from the very people you imagined would be there for you.

This next practice is the same as one you have already been introduced to. Do not be deceived by its simplicity. It is ideal for turbulent times. This is a practice I often use myself. It is what I teach people who are feeling shaky and anxious – after diagnosis; before treatment; or when managing intensity or after difficult news. By doing this practice several times a day, and whenever you need it, you are investing in being more 'grounded'. Experimenting with this for yourself regularly over the next few weeks. This is the only way to discover what it has to offer you.

Your first aid practice is Feet on the Floor, which was introduced to you earlier in this chapter.

Feet on the Floor – with the thread

Feeling the contact of your feet on the ground ... ... just placing your attention down onto the soles of your feet and noticing whatever is there. Exploring the detailed sensations in your toes ... (are they all in contact with your shoes or the floor or do some have more contact than others?) ... ... the balls of the feet (what is the shape of that contact?), and the heels (what is the quality of the contact? how does it feel?). Perhaps feeling the texture of the shoes surrounding the feet ... ... perhaps moving to feel the solid floor beneath you. Noticing the weight of you going down, through your legs onto your feet, onto the floor. Just being curious about all of this – and keep bringing the mind back to the sensations of contact with the floor.

Your thread (see page 16 in Starting Out), and the feel of the bead against your wrist will remind you to come back to your feet on the floor. You can use this practice at any time, whether recently diagnosed or not. It is the basis of much that follows in later 'cancer' practices.

Intention for the 'Month'

We have been exploring the place of intention in the practice of mindfulness. You began by mindfully tasting a raisin – then you were introduced to the Body Scan, the Pause and Feet on the Floor – and you have been taught the First Aid Practice to use with your thread for times of intensity.

Spend some time connecting with your intention this next month – or however long you choose to stay with the practices in this chapter. How might you do this? If you are wearing a thread, you can use it as a reminder. There may be other ways that you can set up to help you remember. Most important of all is to connect with what matters to you – remember your intentions letter – and be ready to begin again and again with your practice.

Practices – *for each 2 week period*

Core Practice   – Body Scan [10+ times]
Short Practices – The Pause [a few times every day]
                      – Feet on the Floor [a few times daily]

Cancer Practice – wearing the thread
                      – First aid practice of Feet on the Floor

Notes

1   Rilke, R.M. (1996)
2   Kabat-Zinn, M., & Kabat-Zinn, J. (2014)
3   With particular appreciation to Christina Feldman.
4   See Appendix 1, also Carlson, et al. (2009)
5   Kornfield, J. (1993)
6   Gawande, A. (2014)
7   Tarrant, J. (1998)
8   Kabat-Zinn, J. (1990, 2013)
9   Moorey, S., & Greer, S. (2012)
10   See soup recipes created by Lee Watson in Appendix 4.

Sometimes

Sometimes things don't go, after all
from bad to worse. Some years, muscadel
faces down frost; green thrives; the crops don't fail,
sometimes a man aims high, and all goes well.

A people sometimes will step back from war;
elect an honest man; decide they care
enough, that they can't leave some stranger poor.
Some men become what they were born for.

Sometimes our best efforts do not go
amiss; sometimes we do as we meant to.
The sun will sometimes melt a field of sorrow
That seemed hard frozen: may it happen for you.

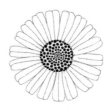

Personal Story

Sarah

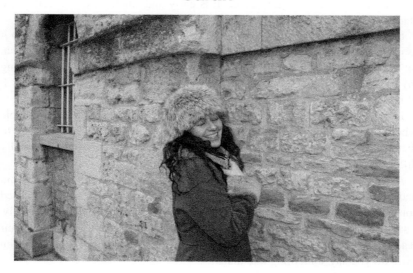

Sarah was 39 when diagnosed with breast cancer. She describes herself as a local North Wales girl, through and through. When her grandfather died, her mother took on the family farm and Sarah bought the little house that her grandfather had lived in. She is carefully doing it up with all its original features, using natural materials. 'This is where my home is and it means the world to me', she told me.

Mindfulness: A Kindly Approach to Being with Cancer, First Edition. Trish Bartley.
© 2017 John Wiley & Sons, Ltd. Published 2017 by John Wiley & Sons, Ltd.
Companion Website: www.wiley.com/go/bartley/mindfulness

Diagnosis

I always remember when it happened. I'd been away and on the way back, I found a message from the hospital, telling me to come in the next day. In the event, I was late for the appointment – would you believe it! I wasn't even sure I was going to make it. There was snow everywhere.

I had been having odd tests with my GP, for the last six months or so. I'd had a biopsy very recently. It was in the back of my mind that something heavy was probably coming. I remember sitting in the waiting room. People started to say, 'She's arrived' and I just thought, 'oh my goodness, tell me now – don't put it off.' They took me into a little room. I don't even remember the name of the consultant, but E, the breast care nurse was there and I could tell she was nervous. They said, 'You've got cancer. It is early and small – but the cells have started replicating.'

I stayed very much in business mode, gathering the facts and dealing with it as if it was a work meeting. I don't think I felt much at all, not even shock. That hit me much, much later – after surgery. When I got back to my house, I rang my boss and texted one of my closest friends. I wasn't ready to deal with much of it yet. I wanted to understand the facts and then I could face it.

I went into work for two days. I remember being in a meeting with people who were having a fit about having to move their desks. I felt like saying to them, 'Do you know I could come to an end?' Their concerns were of a totally different order of things. It was crazy stuff.

After two days, I went home for the weekend. I was dreading telling Mum and Dad. We were sitting round the kitchen table and I don't know if she sensed something because Mum was talking about everything under the sun. Finally, I said, 'Mum, I've got to stop you – I've got cancer.' I can't remember their reaction. I probably didn't tell them very well. I just had to blurt it out. How on earth do you say something like that?

In those early days, I very much equated cancer with death. I told my boyfriend, but I didn't want others to know. I wanted to get through the operation before people started probing. I needed my space. It was a surreal time.

Surgery

Even on the morning of the operation, I came up here to my house. I lit a fire, which is always a very symbolic thing for me to do. It is all connected with this being my home and wanting to take care of it – but it meant I smelt of smoke going into hospital! We had to go in quite early. I have never had to share accommodation – so it felt very strange. Would I be in a huge ward? Would there be talking all the time? In the end, there was only one other lady in the little corner ward with me. It was pleasant enough, but I felt quite trapped.

After surgery and during treatment

I had chemotherapy, then radiotherapy and then Herceptin treatment. During treatment, I freaked out about having to spend time in hospital. I hated the thought of being closed in. So I was keen not to get any colds or bugs. I told my friends that I didn't want visits, but would love them to send me postcards with their news of ordinary life and a favourite picture of themselves. I bought this big notice board and put it by my bed. I spent ages pinning everyone's pictures on it. Nearly every day there would be something in the post. It was lovely.

I was pretty ill with chemo and spent a lot of time in bed feeling rubbish. Mum was brilliant, feeding me tasty things. I remember watching these chicks that I'd bought for her birthday. I would sit in the kitchen looking out of the window, watching them.

My other important occupation was growing trees from seed. I spent a lot of time with plant books, looking at seeds for sale on the Internet, reading up about them, and whether they would they survive the climate here. I learnt how to germinate the seeds with all the temperatures involved. There was a whole industry going on!

It was amazing how quickly I let go of work. All the deadlines and hoo-hah were left behind – something I hadn't done for years. I was back with my parents and they dealt with everything. I was letting myself be looked after. It is interesting. I would lie in bed often feeling quite anxious about being ill, but I remember much more, all the happiness of that time. Isn't it fantastic the way the mind works?

I was conscious of the possibility of cancer coming back and was checking and looking. But what eased my sense of dread was hearing from other people who had come through. Mum had a friend who had treatment a few months before me. She was still there. Other people would tell me about such and such, who had treatment and was fine now. It almost became a body of evidence. This was important, as I like to be rational and logical.

Mindfulness

I got to mindfulness through R, whom I'd had treatment with. We went together on the same course. I was pretty open to it. I found it helpful to approach things in this different way. The way the course was organized suited me quite well, as I like to take time observing things. I enjoyed the practices that were set us – doing things that started off as systematic tasks, but then along the line, realizing that I could change them and do them in my own way. Even now, I do the stretches, reaching for imaginary 'grapes' just above my head. I lie in bed and come to the breath. I loved the movement exercises – and still do. At the time, it was a new activity to learn and maybe a bit of a distraction. Initially the practices and exercises would be isolated events – but as time moved on, I really revelled in them and got a lot from them.

I love seeing the beauty of nature. I appreciated all this before mindfulness, but without realizing how important it was to me. Appreciating the beauty of nature through being mindful is like an affirmation for me of how to approach the world.

Wherever I am, I look carefully at natural things. These are what I see first. This morning, the moon was out and it was bright in the sky – and I felt so lucky to be seeing that. And then whenever I am here, I can always hear the stream. It is always bubbling. It is a perpetual thing – different but always there. I am always walking around the trees and seeing how they are evolving and growing. I buried my dog under one and I talk to her there and feel she is making a beautiful tree.

Post treatment

Chemotherapy finished at the end of July. I used to know all the dates, but now I have to think to remember them. You let it go gently, don't you? I had radio-therapy for three weeks and then Herceptin treatment. One of things that used to worry me was how quickly I would run out of energy.

The house had been broken into during treatment so I was a bit apprehensive about staying here. Dad's dog came back here with me, to protect me. I had heard on the radio about a woman who was bravely fighting for women's rights. I thought to myself – 'well if she could do that, then I'm going to do this' (return to my house). I remember sitting up in bed and writing in my diary about it. This is my home. I was determined to be here for census night. 'I'm back now,' I felt. This place is so important to me.

What matters to me?

Mindfulness is important to me – I do a lot of mindful breathing before I get up in the morning. Time is precious and I don't want to be losing it doing things that are less than precious. I do what I need to do, but I often feel that I want to get on with what is more important.

I am 3+ years post treatment now and I have a much clearer perspective of what matters to me. Illness and treatment has taught me the value of life. I've rediscovered some aunts and uncles and we've become close. I'm glad we've managed this before it is too late. Family networks here in Wales are strong. I think it is to do with the permanence of the land and the softness of the culture.

A message to someone like me

A nurse on the morning of surgery said, 'Keep going at it.' Whenever I got slightly freaked – that little phrase, which sounded quite harsh at the beginning – would really help me. I would think 'Just keep going at it.' You see there was a really laid-back, soft side of me that was just wanting to let go of all responsibility – yet there was another side there as well, that was saying to myself, 'you will go at it, if it should come back.'

I think I gave in to the softer side. I can't ever remember thinking, 'I'm going to fight this. I'm not going to let it get to me.' It was about dealing with it my way. I still check my body and still get scared occasionally, but I could have died in a moment in a car accident and I would never have had the opportunity to do all these things. I've had nearly four really good years now.

I want to enjoy more of this place, and this space. I absolutely love it. I want to learn important skills so I can take care of everything here. It feels good to acknowledge how lucky I am. It hasn't always felt like that. At one point, everyone else seemed to be going off on maternity leave to have babies, whilst I was going off to have cancer. But I feel so fortunate that I have been able to do what I want with my life. I'm so lucky – How many other people have got their granddad's house?!

[translation from Welsh]

Dychwel at Graidd y Graig	Returning to the Root of the Rock
Aros	*Pause*
am anadl,	*a breath,*
Atal adwaith.	*Refrain reaction.*
A dewis.	*Make a choice.*
Clywed y sêr	*Hear the stars*
A gweld curiad y galon,	*And see the beat of the heart,*
Nofio gwynt y storm	*Swim the storm-wind*
A dychwel at graidd y graig.	*And return to the root of the rock.*

Sarah

Chapter 2
Coming Back

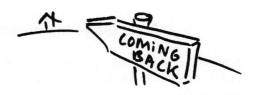

Between stimulus and response, there is a space. In that space is our power to choose our response. In our response, lies our growth and freedom.

Viktor Frankl[1]

We now look at the theme of Coming Back. We develop some understanding of the ways that we struggle and learn some new practices. We review those we have been practicing. We move to another phase of cancer – this time to treatment – and develop practices and approaches targeted to manage treatment and times of waiting.

Mindfulness: A Kindly Approach to Being with Cancer, First Edition. Trish Bartley.
© 2017 John Wiley & Sons, Ltd. Published 2017 by John Wiley & Sons, Ltd.
Companion Website: www.wiley.com/go/bartley/mindfulness

Coming Back – the theme

Coming Back is shorthand for the movement of mind that brings attentive awareness back to the immediacy of this present moment.

Coming Back is at the foundation of the practice of mindfulness. Without it, the mind will continue to do its thing – dwelling on this, obsessing on that, and missing so much of life. Coming Back makes it possible to choose to spend more time aligned with what really matters. This comes into sharp focus after a diagnosis of cancer, when suddenly we experience uncertainty about life and living, maybe for the first time.

Understanding the patterns of suffering

We need to understand more about the ways that we suffer. On one level, we feel we know suffering only too well. But on another, we can only respond to it skilfully, when we understand the mind tendencies to reactivity – and how this causes us difficulty. When we appreciate this more fully, we will be better able to respond mindfully – live with more ease, and focus on what matters most to us.

Patterns of mind

Let us explore some of the patterns of mind that cause us such pain. Remembering that these are patterns that we all share – just by being human.

The 'automatic' wandering of the mind

From your experience of the Body Scan, you will have discovered that the mind rarely stays put – but slides back into the past, *remembering* – or leans forward into the future, *anticipating*. This is what all minds do. 'If you have a mind, it will wander', is repeated by mindfulness teachers around the globe.

Much of the time, the mind is in 'automatic' mode, drifting from this to that, and usually not engaged with what is happening at the time. Researchers confirm that 'a human mind is a wandering mind, and a wandering mind is an unhappy mind.'[2] Mind-wandering seems to be our default mode.

Living in our heads – believing what we think

The development of our brains over the centuries, and way we have been educated, have given us minds that are wonderfully creative, imaginative and able. This is a considerable asset. It helps us to navigate complexity, plan ahead and problem solve. However, we have come to over rely on our intellect and our capacity to think. We dwell in our 'heads' much of the time, believing our thoughts. We have an experience; rush into an explanation for it; and reactions quickly follow.

> Meredith was expecting her son for dinner. He was late and she couldn't reach him on his phone. As time passed, she became more and more anxious, convinced that there had been an accident. An hour later, Sam walked through the door, apologizing. He had met a friend for a drink after work, and his phone was in the car.

Thinking that goes round and round
At times, we slip into a pattern of going over and over something. We might have been trying to push a problem out of mind, but instead find ourselves obsessed with trying to sort it out. There are often no satisfactory answers to be had and we can end up feeling worse and worse – and more stuck, anxious and miserable.

Comparing mind
We have a habit of comparing what we have, with what we would like to have – or what others have – or what we used to have. This can apply to almost anything: possessions, relationships, or even personal qualities. 'If only' is the tell-tale phrase, suggesting that life would be happier and better *if only* I had this, or *if only* I was more like that, or *if only* I had done that.

Wanting, wanting
We are always on the lookout for more of what we want. When you first picked up this book, I wonder if you scanned the pages for poems and interesting looking sections? It is what most of us do. We want quick fixes of enjoyment. Notice how easily we get bored – surfing television channels, turning music on the radio, checking for emails and messages – anything to fill up the gap and offer us some goodies. When we find something that we like – we want to hold onto it – make it ours and need it to stay the same.

Not wanting, avoiding
Whilst working to hold on to what we like, we also try to avoid what we do not like. We push away, tighten and close down to what is difficult and unpleasant. Of course we do. What living being does not? Even a simple creature like a stickleback fish or a housefly reacts by pulling away to being touched. Human patterns of pushing away and avoiding go back to ancient responses to threat.

This is lifesaving when physical danger is imminent. However, in modern everyday life, the very act of pushing away and ignoring things, normal as it is, actually adds to our difficulties, as we will learn.

The added extra of cancer

What we have been exploring so far are universal tendencies that we all share. Simply through being human, we are drawn to seek what we want; avoid what we do not want; and automatically screen out much of the rest.

On top of these tendencies and whatever else is going on, cancer arrives unbidden – deeply shocking, turning lives upside down, and affecting families and entire networks. All the ways that vulnerability commonly shows itself for each person come into stark relief in this new context. On top of the physical challenges, extra layers of suffering are added through the way we react. This is quite normal. We are all susceptible – for the psychological impact of cancer causes more pain and anguish than even the considerable physical burden of illness and treatment.[3]

Let us look through the lens of four specific patterns that are especially relevant to those diagnosed with cancer – at whatever stage they are at.

Trauma
Is widely experienced, as we discussed earlier. The initial diagnosis of cancer can come as such a shock that it can be experienced in a catastrophic way – almost as a death threat. We may feel numbness and disbelief, confusion and loss of meaning. Later, if there is a recurrence, or when waiting for results, follow-up appointments, or on receiving bad news, these spikes of trauma may reappear, bringing with them images or intrusive memories of the initial diagnosis or some previous experience of treatment. Trauma has a shocked frozen quality and it often goes unrecognized.

Sheila saw the look in her mother's eyes when the doctor told them it was cancer. This would come back to haunt her in the weeks and months to come. 'At times I can hardly bring myself to close my eyes to go to sleep. I'm so scared that I might see the expression on her face again', she told me.

Rumination
Is a very common pattern of mind. It is a mechanism that feeds distress. We seem unable to let go of thinking about the painful aspects of getting

cancer, trying to find an answer and discover some way out. The mind goes round and round, over and over, like a 'gramophone record' – often dwelling on how things are now, compared to how things were – or how things might be. We get stuck in judgements, often of ourselves. This way of thinking never dwells in the present – and is always *wanting* things to be different. Rumination can lead to deep suffering. It results in lowering mood and appears never ending.

> George couldn't stop thinking about what had happened to him – the diagnosis; his experience of treatment; why he had got cancer; and most of all whether he would get ill again. He went over it time and time again. Whatever else he was doing, his mind never seemed to stop churning and churning, sometimes leaving him feeling desperately alone and worthless.

Avoidance

Is how we invariably react to painful experiences. It can lead to denial. It might result in us doing things like not using the word 'cancer', or not watching television in case cancer is mentioned. At some level, we are trying to protect ourselves and control the situation, by avoiding emotional pain and the unwanted thoughts that go with it. However, as a strategy, it does not work in the longer term. Reality inevitably intrudes sooner or later, with intense rushes of anxiety. This way of reacting, whilst very human, can increase feelings of distress and leave us feeling very alone and isolated.

> Freda and Ted decided not to tell family and friends about Freda's diagnosis. They did not want to be inundated by visits and phone calls. Ted was firm about this. He didn't even want to talk about it much himself – so Freda was left to manage mostly on her own. When she came on a mindfulness course after treatment, she said it was such a relief to be with people she could share things with.

Distress

Is inevitable and natural. Most people will be distressed at different points in their illness. It is so normal and understandable. Sometimes, when the mood dips, everything can feel pretty hopeless. Waves of tiredness and fatigue seem overwhelming. It can be hard to be motivated to do much at all. Inner judging and negative thoughts add their voices and may result in a tendency to want to withdraw from the world.

A common pattern of distress is one that results in feelings of anxiety and worry. Every ache and pain might be a potential recurrence.

Anne saw her doctor often, ever since her treatment for ovarian cancer. On each occasion, she was sure that the cancer was back. She would spend long periods on the Internet researching symptoms, and getting more and more worried. 'I am convinced every time I find something', she told me. 'My heart pounds; my body is tense; I am sick with fear. Then I am told it is nothing – and I feel a bit better for a while – until some other ache or pain appears, and then it starts all over again.'

Five basic tendencies

If we simplify this further, we see that universally all of us are driven by **wanting** some things and **not wanting** others. Extreme patterns of wanting and not wanting trigger and contribute to overwhelming suffering. Getting cancer, a strong and wholly understandable example of an unwanted experience, can provoke intense feelings of agitation and **worry**, and sometimes **depression** and lethargy. Feeding it all, there is often distressing and sometimes all-consuming **uncertainty** and doubt.

Becoming aware that all of us have these tendencies helps us to respond to them more kindly, and considerably reduces the potential for distress. This is at the very heart of mindfulness practice.

The Approach Of Mindfulness

We now examine why Coming Back is so essential to mindfulness, and what this might offer our struggles and patterns of suffering.

Coming Back to The Body

Through the Body Scan practice, you will have discovered that you have a wandering mind – much like the rest of us! Coming Back is what we call the intentional movement when we choose to bring the mind back to a present moment experience. In this process of Coming Back, there is a strong focus on the body, the breath and physical sensations. Why is this?

The body is usually a good place to come back to, as it does not wander like the mind. It stays reliably close and available to attend to – whether we are sitting, standing, moving or resting. We have different physical sensations all the time – but we can only experience them directly in the presently arising moment. Who can feel yesterday's itch or tomorrow's pain? We might *remember* we had this or that. We may anticipate how it may be tomorrow – but this is not the same as the direct *experience*, which is always happening *now*, in the immediacy of this present moment.

Thoughts on the other hand are always one step removed from immediate experience. They comment *on* the experience and often add an interpretation *of* them, but they are never directly immersed in the experience itself. The mind is agile and can disengage and re-engage attention in short bursts, but it can only deliberately focus on one thing at a time. We seem to be able to do several things at the same time, but many familiar activities are undertaken almost automatically, with very little awareness. By bringing attention to detailed sensations in the body, we offer the mind somewhere to settle.

When we get genuinely curious and engaged with something specific, such as a sensation in the body, the mind is there, right in the experience. Attention, it seems has limited capacity, so if we focus on the body, we cannot at the same time be engaged in thoughts. The mind will wander off at times, but with practice and patience we learn to bring the mind gently back. In time, it almost seems as if the mind starts remembering to come back itself.

So, instead of being stuck in a tangled mass of reactive thoughts and negative emotions, when we bring attention back into physical sensations in the body, we can pause to create a choice about what we might do next. Of course, it takes time to develop this new habit – but even quite early on in your practice, you may notice some beginnings of these changes. The mind learns to settle, on a good day, and we can enjoy what this offers – a glimpse of freedom, a chance to appreciate a new way of being. Little by little, we learn to respond more kindly to what bothers us, and start building new supportive habits.

About half way through his mindfulness course, George was surprised to notice that he needed to file his nails. He had bitten his nails as long as he could remember. Before starting mindfulness, his fingers had been in a terrible state, sometimes bleeding, with the nails bitten down to the quick. Now, they were growing! It was too unusual to be a coincidence. 'Mindfulness seems to be changing the habits of a lifetime', George told me.

Remembering our connection with the physical world

Our first baby steps in this practice of Coming Back start with learning to rely on the body and the breath – which is exactly what you have been doing in the Body Scan. By coming up close to physical sensations, we discourage the mind's usual tendency of jumping from this to that – and give it another place to stand and rest. We are letting the body do its job as the 'container' of experience. We rediscover our connection with the physical world of the senses. We may feel that the body has let us down after a diagnosis of cancer - yet as Jon Kabat-Zinn wisely says:

> *As long as you are breathing, there is more right with you than wrong, no matter how ill or hopeless you may feel.*[4]

Coming back to our senses

When you brought your attention to the raisin, you directly looked, smelled, felt, and tasted it – using all your senses. It may seem an odd thing to do, but by attending carefully to something quite ordinary, we can discover rich insights. Harriet obviously valued this, especially in the context of feeling 'wound up'.

Harriet was surprised by the raisin exercise. She had trained as an artist and thought she knew how 'to focus and think about things.' She phoned me up a few days later. 'I keep thinking about the texture of that raisin' she said, 'I've been so wound up this week with all the hassle of hospital appointments. I've sometimes wondered about holding a raisin again and getting that feeling back. It is hard to explain, but I really knew I was holding that raisin. I could feel the wrinkles and the crevices – and there was nothing else there at all.'

On the face of it, it *is* hard to understand. All she was doing was holding a raisin! But she said that she *knew* she was holding it, and *'there was nothing else there at all'*. It is highly unusual to have nothing else on the mind. Living with cancer is bound to involve troublesome thoughts and feelings. At times, there seems no let-up to the inner cascade of stories tumbling about in the mind.

Here is a little tale that may explain things a bit.

> *Long long ago, two teachers were walking and talking. The younger one asks the older, 'What do you teach your students? They seem to do much better than*

mine.' The older one replies modestly, 'I just teach them to sit, and walk, and lie down.' To which the younger one says, 'but I teach that too.' 'Ah yes', says the wise old teacher, 'but when my students sit, they know *they are sitting; and when they walk, they* know *they are walking; and when they lie down, they* know *they are lying down.'*

Harriet *knew* she was holding the raisin – an apparently significant turn of phrase. For *knowing* the experience, seems to be one of the ways that mindfulness sheds light on experience. This is not an intellectual knowing, but a vivid experiential knowing that fully engages us with the details of what is happening, whilst also pausing the activity of the thinking mind.

Coming to the Breath

Once we come up close to sensations in the body, we encounter the movement of the breath. This dynamic rhythm within the body offers an anchor to the present moment – one that we can always come back to. Like all anchors, it moves and changes – responding to emotional weather and the drifting tides of mood. Coming to the breath is an ancient practice that aligns the *mind* with the *body* – the presently arising moment (*time*) with this very *place*. As we settle into detailed sensations of the rising and falling of the breath, the mind settles. As the mind settles, the breath slows. The process helps us to access calm, without making *that* the goal.

There is much to attend to in the subtle detail of breath. The texture, rhythm, depth, and quality of the breath are all here to explore. We find a whole world to experience, quite different to any other.

Sometimes, when we first pay attention, the breath can become a little shy – as if self-consciously forgetting its natural rhythm. This will ease in time. All that is needed is to give some space to let the breath breathe itself once more. There is no need to control or 'think' the breath. Starting again, letting go and breathing out is a good place to come back to.

Moving up close to the breath, seeing if you can be there at the very moment that the breath first breathes in. There is a lift in the breath and it is a pity to rush it. There is magic in simply waiting patiently – experiencing the moment when the breath itself, breathes in. It is extraordinary how much experience is there to discover just by bringing a fresh curiosity to something we know so well.

Peter came to love being with his breath. When talking about this, he put his hand down beside him. 'It is like my old dog, always with me, close by.'

As if for the first time – bringing curiosity to the ordinary

In the beginner's mind there are many possibilities, in the expert's there are few.[5]

This brings Rilke's river poem to mind.[6] (We looked at this at the start of the Intention chapter.) He wanted to flow like a river … *'the way it is with children'.* When we experience things that are familiar and ordinary *as if for the first time*, fresh and immediate, it completely changes the experience. We move from automatic to present; perhaps from irritation to calm; maybe even from boredom to the possibility of wonder.

If I could have waved a fairy wand at your birth and wished upon you just one gift, it would not have been beauty or riches or a long life; it would have been the gift of wonder.[7]

I have a long journey to get to work. The road goes past lovely mountains and coastline, yet I can sometimes resent having so far to drive. When I remember to come back and make the journey *as if for the first time,* I see new detail every time – resentment long forgotten.

Alternative Anchors

Sometimes, for some people, it can be wise to find another place to come back to.

> Anne, a gentle lady, had been cleared of lung cancer, but found it hard to accept that she had survived when so many had not. Miserable and depressed, sleeping badly, and fiercely self-critical, she said she felt she deserved for the cancer to return. Happily, it didn't. When she started mindfulness, she found it difficult to be with the breath. It was too close to illness and treatment. Instead, she discovered the value of hearing sounds. This is what she came back to. Little by little, as her mind became steadier, she learned to be more kind to herself. 'Coming back to the sounds around me has made all the difference', she told me.

Cultivating kindly awareness

I remember being asked whether the activity of a burglar could be described as mindful. This really caught my attention. We can easily imagine a burglar creeping about a house – vigilant and aware of every sound, the position of each piece of furniture, highly alert to the possibility of needing to react rapidly. The burglar is paying careful attention. Yet is he mindful? And if not, what is missing?

Mindfulness has many qualities. It certainly does need us to 'pay attention', though this always sounds a bit like a schoolroom injunction! However, there is a quality in mindful attention that the burglar does not have.

Mindfulness asks us to relate to experience in a friendly way. We form an intention to bring the mind back to the body *gently*. Paying attention, without this, can be tight and fixed – like the burglar. Kindliness and friendliness invite a quality of heart. Wise response is very different to our habitual tendency to judge and criticize.

Mindfulness as practice

Mindfulness is often compared to playing a musical instrument, or to developing a creative skill. Even with lots of natural talent, it still takes years of practice to produce a lovely sound or create a beautiful work of art. So it is with mindfulness. This is not a quality that we acquire in a moment. It is a rich cultivation that develops and matures over a lifetime. There will always be more to learn and explore. Mindfulness, which is warmly befriending, can accompany us to our very last breath – and enrich our lives all the way to that point. There are few things that can offer this much.

> *The present is the only time that any of us have to be alive – to know anything ... to act – to change – to heal.*[4]

Summary

Through the practice of connecting to sensations in the body and the breath, we learn to 'come back' to ourselves.

Some key reminders:

- Becoming aware of detailed physical sensation – using all *the senses* – coming back to the body and the breath.
- Being curious about the experience *as if for the first time* – especially with ordinary everyday things.
- Seeing if it is possible to *befriend* the breath, the body, and whatever is happening.
- Becoming aware of the experience and *knowing* that you are

Got Up Mindfully This Morning

Got up mindfully this morning,
my mind was here and there,
but I was aware
til the end of the day.

Ruth (16)

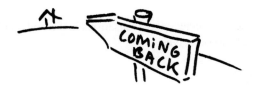

Practices And Approaches

This immediacy of knowing – right now – of the breath, a sound, some movement, points to the innate wakefulness of our minds. We learn to become familiar with it, and trust it ... It is all within us: we are what we are looking for.

Joseph Goldstein[8]

We know a bit more now about what makes us suffer. We have also learned that coming back to mindfulness can interrupt the patterns that create our suffering. Now, we learn to put this into practice.

Overview

In this section we look at:

- Some new practices – core and short ones.
- Reviewing the practices you have been following.
- An exercise and some approaches that help you further develop your understanding of how the mind reacts in the context of cancer.

New Practices

Core Practice	– Mindful Walking (formal and informal)
Short Practices	– Standing in Mountain
	– Coming to the Breath

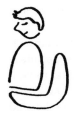

Core Practice

Mindful movement

Now that you are more familiar with sensations in the body when you are still, through the Body Scan practice – we move on to explore awareness of the body in movement. We are learning to come back to the body, in all its different modes – and as we do, we find subtle differences day-by-day, and moment-by-moment. For example, I notice that my limbs and joints feel easier when I walk after a good nights sleep. I take a similar route most days, yet I notice different sensations in my body and different things around me, every time.

When setting out on these movement practices, we cultivate an intention to become aware of the details of our experience – rather than general impressions. We are deliberating developing the capacity to be precise and aware, moving up close to what we notice.

Mindful Walking

Normally, we walk for a purpose – to get somewhere; to take exercise; to spend time with someone. We rarely walk just to walk.

While walking, the attention usually drifts from one thing to another. An appealing storyline appears in the mind – and we linger there. An unpleasant smell wafts across – and we crinkle the nose. We are usually a long way from awareness of the body, (unless thinking about a sensation) – and probably unaware of what is around us – except in a flickering, random way.

We can change this by turning the walking into an opportunity to practice Coming Back. Walking is wonderfully flexible and accessible. We can do it almost anywhere – and it has many possibilities. This makes walking practice suitable for almost all of us[9] – even for very short periods, for those with discomfort in the feet or body.

'Slow' mindful walking – the way to begin

A traditional form of walking practice involves slowing the process down to allow us to notice more. It can feel a bit unnatural at the beginning – but it is worth persevering. It offers us a way of bringing attention to very detailed sensations. This is a valuable skill to acquire in our mindfulness repertoire, and is very different to our usual way of doing things.

There is a guided practice on the website. Later when you are familiar with it, you can leave the recording behind and follow your own 'freestyle' practice – guiding yourself as you walk. If mindful walking is unfamiliar to you, follow the practice at least 10–15 times, or however many times you feel you need it, in order to build momentum in Coming Back and exploring detailed sensations.

Mindful walking – guidance

1 *Walking along a 'track'*
Finding somewhere – in the house, garden or yard, where you will not be disturbed or overlooked – where you can walk on the flat, in a straight line for 10 or 20 paces. The point of the practice is not to go anywhere, but just to be with the experience of walking.

2 *Standing in Mountain (as guided on the website practice)*
We start by placing attention into the contact of the feet as they rest on the floor… spending a little time with this … really feeling the contact points in toes … balls of the feet … and heels at the back … and feeling the firmness of the ground or the floor beneath you …. Then moving attention up the legs, checking that the knees are soft and not locked … … the pelvis is slightly tucked …. Standing tall, feeling the spine rising up out of the pelvis, up though the back … … and into the shoulders, allowing them to be down … … and following the passage of the spine up into the neck … slightly tucking the chin, so that there is a little stretch up the back of the neck … … and extending up through the middle of the head to the top of the back of the crown of the head. Standing like a mountain … rooted and grounded, tall and dignified … … abiding presence – breathing mountain.

3 *Starting to walk*
After fully experiencing this sense of 'mountain' standing, forming the intention to move.

Transferring the weight onto your right foot so that your left foot whilst still on the ground, holds almost no weight ... (how does that feel? – just noticing sensations) ... ... then when you are ready, lifting your left foot and moving it a little way until it comes to rest on the ground ... ... present at the footfall, your attention really there as you place the foot on the ground ... ... feeling the transfer of weight onto the left foot ... and then repeating the process with the right foot ... lifting ... moving ... placing ... present each time at the footfall.

You can repeat 'lifting, moving, placing' internally to yourself as you practice this. It helps to remember to come back to the sensations in the feet and legs.

4 **Pausing at the end of each track**
As you come to the end of each track, you pause before turning around ... ... and come back to feeling your feet on the floor ... ... and then coming to your breath, feeling the movement of the breath breathing ... . Just standing and being aware of standing and of breathing. Sometimes you might want to say to yourself: 'Here – Now.'

Then when you are ready, slowly turning yourself around to face the other way, noticing the sensations of turning as you do – and then setting off the other way, mindfully walking.

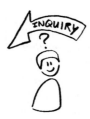

Reflective inquiry of the walking practice

1   What did you notice about some aspect of that experience of walking – in general/in detail?

> Barbara noticed the way her heel came down as she walked. For some moments, she was able to become aware of the different parts of her feet and the particular sensations as they came in contact with the floor.

2   How was that for you?

> Jenny found mindful walking to be irritatingly slow. She said that her mind wandered a lot, and she found herself longing for the practice to end. When she mentioned this in the group, her teacher asked if anyone else had noticed this, and a number of people nodded in agreement.

3   What do you make of that, if anything?

> Barbara noticed that when she was engaged in the detailed experience of walking, her mind wandered less. She felt more settled and this was a pleasant feeling.

> Jenny realized that she was not on her own in finding mindful walking irritating. Her experience was different to Barbara's, and that was ok.

Remember that we are not trying to create any special feelings as a result of practice – we are simply learning to bring awareness to the body as it moves, and noticing how that is. Every time we practice, the experience will be different. We tend to assume that a practice is 'better' or 'worse' than another. We all have preferences, but there is value in following the practice as best we can, bringing curiosity and kindly attention to whatever our experience is – whether pleasant or unpleasant and whatever effect is felt.

Practice mindful walking at least 10 times over the next two weeks – either using the guided practice – or on your own for 10 minutes or more. Reflecting on your experience after the practice using the reflective inquiry process or your own questions.

Additional Practice Ideas

This is included for those with some existing experience of mindfulness – or after mindful walking is established.

Further ideas for walking practices

- Up the stairs, in the supermarket, on the way to the car, moving around the kitchen – i.e. everyday 'ordinary' walking.
- At work – along corridors (especially when busy), between desk and printer, walking to meetings.
- Planned walks – in the countryside, the park, around the garden, down the street.
- Whenever you walk, bring awareness to the contact of your feet with the floor, for a few moments – or longer, if you want.

Added ingredients to walks, after the core practice is established

- SIGHTS – near and far – colour, shape, different greens/blues/yellows, etc. – things moving/things that are still.
- SOUNDS – wind, clothing, feet on ground, birdsong, traffic sounds.
- TEXTURES – smooth/rough – thin/thick – wet/dry.
- WHOLE BODY – the whole body moving – and awareness of the space around you.

Coming back to your footfall every now and again – stopping and pausing to notice (*What is going on for me right now?*) – tracking the rhythm of breathing – your levels of tiredness/energy – and maybe your mood.

Additional or optional practice

Mindful stretching

On the website, there is also a simple mindful stretching practice. This can be adapted in whatever way is best for you:

- sitting in a upright chair
- standing
- or sitting in a comfortable chair with eyes closed imagining you are doing the stretches.

Deciding what might be best in advance – and then choosing how much and how long to hold the stretches.

Choosing

You can vary your mindful movement practice, day-by-day, if you want to. Perhaps you might follow the stretches one day, and then do the walking practice the next. Or you can choose what to practice on the day, depending on how you feel and what you need.

Joan had spent a happy, but exhausting, day with her grandchildren. The next day, she was tempted to give her practice a miss – but she was also keen to keep going if she could. She decided to do a few stretches. 'I was tired, but my body actually seemed to enjoy stretching. I deliberately did it very gently and not for too long. I was pleased that I had', she said.

Your own movement practice

You may have your own personal Yoga, Qi Gong, or other movement practice. It might be perfect to continue with this – perhaps adapting it in small ways.

The key shift may be in changing the intention of your practice right at the start. Instead of seeking to improve tone or flexibility, to extend and develop the poses, or learn a routine, get fit and so on – you might translate your intention to do your movement practice very mindfully. The change might seem tiny – but by bringing a mindful perspective to the forefront of your practice, you may discover things within your experience that offer you rich insight in other contexts.

You might experiment by including the following components in your practice:

- Pausing and noticing what is going on for you.
- Using the breath to breathe into any intensity.
- Moving your mind right into the stretch or intensity and making choices, moment by moment, about how long to hold the pose or movement.
- Bringing compassion and a gentle attitude to your body as you move.
- Coming Back over and over to sensations in the body.

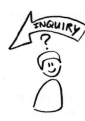

Reflective inquiry

- What did you notice about some aspect of that practice – in general/in detail?
- How was that for you?
- What do you make of that, if anything?

Using the same questions to reflect for a few moments each time you practice. It does not need to take long, but inquiring of your practice will serve to develop and deepen your learning. It will help you to link your experience of practice and apply this into your everyday life choices.

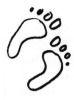

Short Practices

These short practices are really important. They give you a way of threading mindfulness into everyday life, to use wherever you are, and with whatever feeling, thought or situation might arise.

Standing In Mountain

This short practice is just the same as the start of the walking practice. This is a simple thing to do, standing at the window, outside somewhere, in the office, anywhere. It enables you to come directly into the body, standing tall with the feet on the floor, feeling grounded, stable and 'earthed'.

 Standing in mountain

We start by placing attention into the contact of the feet on the floor ... ... spending a little time with this ... really feeling the contact points in toes ... balls of the feet ... and heels at the back ... and feeling the firmness of the ground or the floor beneath you ... ... then moving attention up the legs, checking that the knees are soft and not locked ... ... the pelvis is slightly tucked ... ... and standing tall, feeling the spine rising up out of the pelvis, up though the back ... ... and into the shoulders, allowing them to be down ... ... and following the passage of the spine up into the neck ... slightly tucking the chin, so that there is a little stretch up the back of the neck ... ... and extending up through the middle of the head to the top of the back of the crown of the head. Standing like a mountain ... rooted and grounded, tall and dignified ... abiding.

Many people use this when going through anxious times.

> Eleanor had to have a very tough course of treatment in a large hospital away from home. She was dreading it, but it was her best chance of stopping the spread of cancer. Of all the practices she had learnt, Standing in Mountain was her favourite. Whenever she felt scared or anxious, she would stand up and do the practice, really focusing on the feel of her feet on the floor – and the solid of the ground beneath her. She would finish by coming to the breath at the end. Some days she would need to do this many, many times. 'It holds me together', she said, 'and helps me quite literally keep my feet on the ground.'

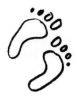

Coming to the Breath

Awareness of the breath can be a steadying resource. It acts as an anchor to come back to – a place of safety – enabling us to *step out of* 'mindlessness', where the mind wanders to unhelpful places – and *step into* present awareness. Coming to the Breath is very simple and effective – for the breath is always here in the body to come back to.

Coming to the Breath

You start by shifting position to become aware of your feet on the floor ... the feel of your body in contact with the chair ... holding you. Weight going down ... Then, when you are ready, connecting with a sense of your spine rising up through the body, holding you upright ... tall ... dignified ... Height going up.

Becoming aware of the fact that you are breathing ... Letting the breath breathe itself – not interfering with it in any way ... simply feeling the sensations of the breath deep within the body.

If at any point, you notice that your mind has wandered away from the breath ... into thinking, or distracted by a sound, or perhaps drawn to a sensation in the body, remembering that this is not a problem – it is what minds do ... And as soon as you realize that you have wandered away, gently coming back to the anchor of the breath ... to the sensations of the waves of the breath breathing in, and breathing out.

Everyday routine activities

You can practice very simply by bringing mindful awareness to any activity. There are many examples of routine activities that you could choose from. Here are some that others have used:

- Having a shower – *smell, contact, sound, movement, feeling.*
- Waiting for the kettle to boil – *standing with awareness, listening.*
- Booting up the computer – *pausing, breathing, feet on the floor.*
- Doing the washing up – *smell, feel, sound.*
- Making the bed – *touch, movement, sight.*
- Getting into bed – *feeling, contact, (smell of clean sheets).*

Paul was sitting in the oncology waiting room the other day and greeted me as I walked past. He told me that he often thinks of me when he mindfully cleans his teeth! 'If I manage nothing else when I'm busy', he told me, 'At least I am mindful a few times a day when I scrub my teeth!'

Janet regularly has a mindful shower – smelling the soap or shower gel hearing the water, feeling it on the skin, feeling the contact beneath her feet, etc. It is a practice she loves. 'It sets me up for the day', she said.

Julia has a favourite practice. She watches and listens to the bubbles in her gin and tonic!

Dick enjoys his food. He is especially fond of curry. After his first mindfulness session, he went to his favourite Indian restaurant and ordered his favourite dish to take home. He told us about this the following week in class. 'Usually I just shovel it in', he said, demonstrating this with his hands, 'This time, I tasted every mouthful. It was really delicious!'

Home Practice Review

We now reflect on the practices that you have been doing these last weeks. We start with the Body Scan and move on to the two short practices of The Pause and Feet on the Floor.

Body Scan – the Core Practice

What are you noticing? Of course, every time will be different, and there will be many experiences in each practice. Allowing for that – let us reflect on your practices, using similar questions to before.

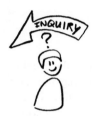

Reflective inquiry

- What have you noticed about your experience of practicing the Body Scan over this time?
- How has that been for you?
- What do you make of that, if anything?

Margaret noticed that she has started to enjoy the Body Scan. 'At first I found it difficult to stay put for that length of time. There were so many other things I needed to do', she told me. But as the time passed, she noticed some benefit. 'Even if I slept through parts of it, when I got to the end, I felt that I had made good use of that time. I think it is helping me feel a bit steadier generally', she finished.

If you prefer – you can reflect internally or in your notebook:

What general differences have I noticed, compared to when I started?

Some common issues in the body scan

Staying awake

> Chris seemed a bit downhearted. 'Every time I do the body scan, I fall asleep.' Chris had been sleeping badly for ages, so although he enjoyed the rest – he wanted to experience the whole practice. 'I've tried doing it first thing in the morning', he said. 'This is only any help if I've had a reasonable night's sleep.' What helped the most, he discovered, was his intention to stay awake. 'I connect with wanting to do the practice with as much awareness as possible. And I commit myself to that as the practice starts. It sounds so simple, but it seems to help.'

Mind wandering

During the practice, we will often find ourselves *thinking* – planning the evening meal; what to say to somebody; remembering some event during the day; caught up in a daydream. We may be drawn to some *sensation* in the body – perhaps an itch or some restlessness. As best we can, we simply notice and come back to wherever we have got to in the practice. We are training the 'coming back muscle'. Sometimes, we have to come back to the body over and over. This *is* the practice.

No right way

It is easy to imagine that a 'good' practice is when the mind is clear and still and stays focused – and a 'bad' practice is when the mind is wandering a lot, or very sleepy. This is not so. Simply practicing coming back and realising the habits of mind, without judging them, is probably the most helpful practice we can have. We are learning to be with things as they are, from moment to moment. We are learning that we are much like everyone else – with a mind that wanders.

Cultivating kindness

As we bring awareness to the body, we may come across intense sensations, or find parts of the body that hold agitation, tightness or heaviness. As best we can, we are learning to relate to these experiences without struggle. Our aim is not to get rid of them (however appealing that sounds). Mindful attention is kindly, so we meet the affected area with as much care as we can, being guided by what feels do-able. Our intention is to befriend pain and anxiety, whenever we can, especially within an area of treatment. This takes courage and needs time and patience. Could you begin by approaching the part of the body involved, as if it was a small wounded animal, or a hurt child?

Developing precise attention – and letting go

The Body Scan is training the mind to focus in on detail. At times we move up close to somewhere in the body, like the toe or the knee. We explore the detail of the sensation there. Then, at another times, we widen the beam of attention to take in a bigger area, such as the whole foot, or the trunk of the body. We are developing the mind's capacity to be both one pointed and then to be wide focused.

Now and then, we deliberately let go of an area of attention, such as the left leg – and move to another area and focus on that, such as the right foot. In this way, we are exercising the 'attentional muscle', learning how to purposely direct the attention. The breath helps us here, particularly when we use an imaginary breath as the vehicle for awareness – travelling down one side of the body to breathe into the foot or the leg, and travelling back up to breathe out of the nose or mouth.

Through the Body Scan, we learn to be more precise in the way we move, change, let go, and widen the attention. It is a bit like going to the gym to exercise the body. Here we are training the mind.

The role of intention

However fruitful this training can be, there are probably times when we do not feel like doing it. We may be busy, feel bored, resistant, or just not sufficiently motivated to keep going. If this becomes a pattern, it is wise to come back to your intention.

Perhaps you might revisit the first chapter and remember why you embarked on this approach. Look at what you wrote about what really mattered to you. Do you want to continue? Do you have any sense of benefitting from what you have done thus far? Is it a pattern for you to tail off on things that you start? If the answer is yes to these questions – then simply begin again, starting now. No need to give yourself a bad time or judge yourself harshly. We all have times when we need to remember what we intended and begin again. We can always do that with mindfulness.

Make a decision now when you will next practice and how often you intend to practice this week – and then stick to it, as best you can!

Short practices review

These practices only take a few seconds, yet they are hard to remember. We can set up reminders. For example, you can put coloured sticky dots on the mirror, computer, tablet, steering wheel, etc. You might consider setting up reminders on your phone, perhaps using a mindful bell app, if that appeals to you! It really is essential to find ways to establish these practices, almost as a habit to come back to – there whenever and wherever we need them.

1 **Feet on the Floor**
2 **The Pause**

Reflective inquiry of the short practices

- What have you noticed about your experience of practicing Feet on the Floor and the Pause over this time?
- How has that been for you?
- What do you make of that, if anything?

Simon described his struggle to remember the Pause. 'Feet on the Floor was much easier for me somehow', he said. 'I enjoyed coming back to my feet and could feel some benefit in being more grounded. But I don't get the point of doing a Pause. Even when I remember it, I'm not sure what I'm meant to be doing.'

In contrast, Maria really got into the Pause. 'It helps me to interrupt things and notice what's happening. I think I might even be slowing down a bit', she said.

If you prefer – you can reflect in your journal:

What general differences have I noticed, having practiced these two short practices?

Approaching And Understanding Experience

Thoughts And Feelings

This is a central exercise in this approach, and is taken from standard cognitive therapy practice.

Walking down the street[10]

You can follow the opening part of the exercise from the website. It goes as follows:

'I invite you now to imagine a short scenario that I will describe. Your task is simply to follow the instructions, if that is okay for you and see what your reaction is at the end. You'll be asked to answer some questions in a certain order and then to record your answers. Please answer the first question before going on to read or answer the second. You will need to have your notebook and a pen to hand before you start. The whole exercise is quite short and will only take a few minutes.'

'You are walking down the street, in your own town or shopping area … … On the other side of the road, you see a friend … … You smile and wave … … but your friend doesn't seem to notice and keeps on walking, and is soon out of sight … …

Pausing to notice your reactions – and asking yourself what is going on for me right now?'

How do you feel?

Using your journal to jot down your responses to this question, drawing out any feelings or emotions as a result of this imaginary experience – or just have that in mind. Now turn to the next questions.

What do you think happened?

What was the story that you were telling yourself? For example, did your friend see you?

You might want to organize your page in the following way.

A. Walking down the street

B. Thoughts	C. Feelings
Your thoughts about what happened – the story ...	What you were left with?

Before we look at this further, I will share some responses from the current group.

A. Walking down the street

B. Thoughts	C. Feelings
*The friend didn't see me, but others did!	Silly
*I wanted to tell her my news	Regret
*He was ignoring me	Annoyed
*I was invisible to her	Sad
*'What have I done?' (she saw me)	Worried
'Be like that then'	Angry

If you take a piece of paper and cover over the words on the left-hand **B** column – you have the title **A** across the top, and the **C** column down on the right. Can you see that this is our usual experience? Something happens – and we quickly have feelings about it.

We may be unaware of the story that we have constructed around it (column B). When we look at the list the current group made, we see that each feeling was the natural consequence of each assumption. For example, I *would* feel sad, if my friend saw me and ignored me. 'I was invisible to her', would be my interpretation.

Our problem is two-fold.

1   We may be unaware of the interpretations and assumptions that we make. They often lie just beneath the surface of our awareness.
2   Yet the way we interpret an event (the story we construct around it) directly results in how we feel about it.

Thoughts Are Not Facts

It is not so much the situation itself but the meaning that we give to it that leads to how we react.

Our interpretations are based on a wide variety of influences such as personal history, context, previous experience and even quite random thoughts.

These reactions often follow old stories and patterns – along automatic grooves in the mind.

There is often no evidence for our thoughts. They are just part of an internal commentary that is being constructed much of the time. An event happens – we jump to conclusions – yet everyone has their own perspective. The mind will always generate meanings and interpretations.

We can affirm the wisdom of the statement:

THOUGHTS ARE NOT FACTS
(even those that say that they are)

The influence of mood

Jo gets up after a poor night's sleep. She is feeling anxious about the day ahead. A letter arrives in the post from the hospital with an unexpected appointment with her oncologist

How might Jo feel? What internal stories might be running that influence her reaction to the letter?

Derek has recently started a new relationship. He wakes up feeling happy, remembering that he is seeing his girlfriend later that day. A letter arrives in the post from the hospital with an unexpected appointment with his oncologist.

How might Derek feel? What internal stories might be running that influence his reaction to the letter?

Mood has a strong influence on how we react. As we can see from the examples above, the same event happening when we are in one mood may lead to quite different feelings when we are in another. Additionally, how we react may continue to affect our mood for some time to come. If we can notice what is happening and spot the links between events, mood and the internal stories we tell ourselves, we are less likely to be sucked into them.

The Pause and other short practices help us to slow down and stay in touch with physical sensations, thoughts and feelings. We may not catch the troublesome reactions straight away, but even if we manage to catch them later, it helps us to choose our response. This can have a significant impact on reducing patterns of anxiety and low mood.

Summary – thoughts are not facts

$$A \; (situation) + B \; (thoughts) = C \; (emotions)$$

We find ourselves in a situation (A) that results in feeling an emotion (C). Just under the surface of awareness are the automatic thoughts, (B), which interpret what has happened. These come in the form of an internal commentary, a bit like background noise, that tend to tell the same stories about the world and our part in it. This results in our reactions and feelings – feeding patterns of anxiety and low mood.

Mapping The Experience

Sometimes, we can become overwhelmed by something that in hindsight does not seem so significant. By becoming aware of the way that we interpret events, we can begin to disentangle our overall experience. The Blob helps us to do this.

The Blob[11]

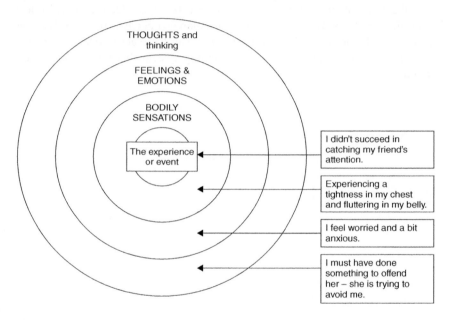

The First Ring – brings us to notice the physical sensations. Increasingly, we are learning to come back to the body and what it is telling us.

The Second Ring – involves emotions or feelings, which may just be a vague sense of something pleasant, unpleasant or neither one nor the other.

The Third Ring – draws out the thoughts, interpretations or stories we are telling ourselves about the event or experience - the inner commentary.

Later we can include a fourth circle that relates to what we do – and how we behave – as a result of something happening.

Many of us find it difficult to tell thoughts from feelings. The Blob helps us to do this. By teasing out the different strands of our experience, we can get into the practice of noticing feelings (which come quickly and always have an effect in the body) and thoughts (which are more like a commentary or a picture about what has happened). All these layers are interconnected. We have a thought, which generates a feeling, which produces a sensation in the body. Sometimes the order seems to differ, but whatever the order, we are learning to come back to the body, as a first response.

A useful metaphor is that of a telephone exchange, overflowing with different coloured wires. Seen from the outside, it looks like a gigantic mess. Knowing how to identify the different colours and their patterns, phone engineers can make sense of the whole thing. In the same way, once we learn how to recognize the different dimensions of our experience, (thoughts, feelings and physical sensations in the body), we can start to disentangle ourselves from our familiar patterns and storylines. We can change the way we react to events, and free ourselves from an apparently ever expanding system that threatens to overwhelm us.

Pleasant Experiences

Over the next month or so, in the interests of noticing what we often miss – you are invited to pay special attention to pleasant experiences.

This might be something that you enjoy, or find beautiful, or in any way experience as pleasurable. It might be a significant experience, or something very small and ordinary – a child's smile; a flower in the garden; a kind remark; a patch of sunlight; a birdsong. Noticing something every day that is pleasant or enjoyable – and pausing to give it your attention for a moment or two.

You can use The Blob to record these pleasant experiences. You can draw a blob yourself – and then fill it in. Some people talk about 'blobbing' their experience. They like mapping the different layers of what is happening.

Paying attention to the lovely

When we are going through tough times, we can forget to notice the flowers in spring, or the colours of autumn. We may screen out the sound of birdsong. We are so busy moving on to the next thing, or internally preoccupied with some storyline, or some troublesome emotion – that we tend to lose much of what goes on around us.

Things change so quickly. A little bud opens into a flower in such a short time, yet if we forget to notice, we will miss it entirely and the flower will have died before we know it.

Spring is in full swing here. The birds are busy feeding their young. There is a raven's nest high in one of the fir trees. When the parent birds land to bring food to the young, they appear huge against the sky – and their raven chicks make a racket as they greet the arrival of their next meal. I sometimes just stand and listen and watch.

Can you go to the window? What can you see? Even if there is nothing special in sight, can you find something to pay attention to? Go out into the garden, or walk to the park, just for the purpose of noticing something that is lovely. Nature is a great ally here.

Home Practice For Coming Back

Core Practice	– Mindful Walking/Mindful Stretching (or both) *Alternating with Body Scan if you want*
Short Practices	– Standing in Mountain – Coming to the Breath – Everyday routine activity *Continuing with The Pause and Feet on the Floor*
Pleasant Experiences	– Noticing a pleasant experience every day and recording it using the Blob or your journal

Intention for this month

Thoughts are not Facts ... ... Noticing the ways that we interpret events.

We now look at another experience of cancer – this time of treatment. We use the skills and learning we have been gathering to bring to experiences that challenge us.

The Experience Of Cancer

Treatment

The gap between diagnosis and treatment is hopefully short, yet this time can feel hectic. There are appointments to attend, decisions to make, previous commitments to unmake, and a vast range of experience to process. It is not surprising if you feel overwhelmed.

Information will come from many sources. You may be hungry for facts and figures, desperate to get the 'ground' back under your feet. Or you may be resistant to know too much, for fear of what may emerge. At the beginning, it may not be easy to determine what is relevant and what is not. There is a risk of becoming even more anxious, (yet most of us do it) as we trawl the Internet for clues as to what is in store. Some information you find on the net will be well researched. Some will be based on subjective experience, which may or may not apply to you – and which may leave you feeling alarmed.

Making decisions about treatment options is challenging. On the one hand, we want to be told what to do. 'The doctor knows best', is very reassuring if we trust him or her. On the other hand, we want to understand what is involved in the decisions, yet we know so little about the implications. Some physicians are much more skilled than others in communicating with their patients – yet this may not necessarily reflect their skills in treating cancer. Hopefully we have a team of medical professionals and can access a range of support, but this may not always be the case.

Becoming a patient in the medical system can leave us feeling young and dependent. We may feel sad and angry at times – and appreciative, and even quite calm at others. It is quite normal to have strong feelings and find your emotions move in different directions at different times. Soon after diagnosis, life may feel rather special and dramatic, which can buoy us up for a while – but as time passes, this generally fades and the reality of having cancer seems to seep into life – perhaps feeling more like a marathon than a starring role.

Things may prove to be different from what we might expect. There are bound to be challenges – but there are also extraordinary developments in the treatment of cancer, and many opportunities to experience kindness. At first, it is all very new and strange. We go on a steep learning curve as patients, possibly finishing up feeling like something of an expert in our particular type, stage, and treatment of cancer.

Staying positive, resourceful and kindly towards your experience is an intention that is worth sustaining – whilst being open to letting in and being nurtured by the support, love and kindness that is offered by friends, family, and medical professionals. You do not have to do this on your own – whatever your personal situation.

The following suggestions come from people who have been through treatment themselves:

- keeping an open mind.
- remembering that everyone's experience is different (even if there are some common side-effects).
- approaching treatment with a positive attitude that it will be helpful.
- resourcing yourself as best you can, with mindfulness practices and whatever other support is helpful.
- taking in people's kindness.

We now move on to share some specific short practices – for waiting and for treatment. They are all available to download from the book's website. We use the thread to help remind you of these practices.

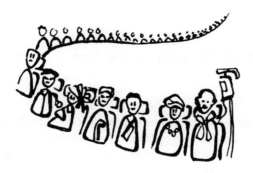

Waiting

 We will often find ourselves *waiting*. There will be waiting at home for results, news, appointments, and decisions. We will sit waiting in hospitals, clinics, consulting rooms, and surgeries. We will join queues of others, waiting for X-rays, scans, medicines and blood tests. Waiting is part and parcel of being a 'patient' and having cancer. Some waiting may be boring and tedious. Often, we wait feeling anxious and afraid, with others who probably feel similarly.

Come to the hospital or clinic prepared to wait - with a book to hand (maybe this one), your notebook, a pen, a bottle of water, and loads of patience.

Waiting mindfully

A waiting practice is described below followed by two additional practices. It is best to follow the key practice first, until you are very familiar with it. It will not take you long, if you have been following the short practices thus far. Eventually you may choose to combine the basic practice with one or both additional ones. On the other hand, you may prefer to find your own way of waiting. Be creative. Practice what works best. You are the expert.

Mindful waiting practice

Start by practicing **The Pause** *with your eyes open. Stopping and asking yourself, 'How am I feeling right now?' or 'What is going on for me right now?'... ... ... taking care not to get carried away by your inner commentary, but focusing on noticing your direct experience ... ... Then, bringing attention to your* **Feet on the Floor** *... feeling the contact between the toes, balls of the feet, and heels with your shoes and the floor beneath ... ... And when the mind wanders, see if you can gently come back to your feet on the floor... ... and widen to include your body and the contact with the seat.*

Additonal Practice Ideas

Two additional practices follow for those with some existing practice of mindfulness. The first has been developed for waiting with *uncertainty*. The second takes this further by holding *anxiety* in a kindly way.

 Waiting and breathing with[12]

Following the **Waiting Practice** of The Pause and Feet on the Floor ... ... *and then expanding to include the contact of your body with what you are sitting on ... ... then widening further to include your breath breathing in your body ... ... with your eyes open,* **Breathing With** *whatever is happening around you and within you ... ... having some awareness on your feet on the floor and some awareness on your breath breathing.*

Waiting with kindness[13]

*Follow the **Waiting Practice** of the Pause and Feet on the Floor ......and then looking around at the others waiting with you, and internally offering them your **Kindly Good Wishes**.......and repeating one or more of the kindness phrases silently and internally, if you would like to:*

'May you be well, in the midst of treatment',
'May you be peaceful, in the midst of uncertainty,
'May you be safe and protected, even in the midst of fear.'

Choosing a phrase to suit you and gently repeating it internally whenever you are aware of feeling anxious ... ...

It may seem strange to offer kindly phrases to others, whenever you are aware of feeling anxious yourself. Of course, you can also offer these phrases to yourself or to everyone waiting (including you). However, it helps to start by choosing someone specifically who you feel drawn to, and internally wishing kindness to them. Later you can expand this further to include yourself and others as well.

When waiting, there is often a lot going on internally, and probably on the outside around you too. So it is wise to keep your waiting practice simple and straightforward.

Treatment

 Cancer treatment is changing all the time, improving in effectiveness, grounded by research, and often with reduced side effects. Having said that, many treatments are still challenging and arduous. Remember to use your waiting practices before treatment, and mixing and matching practices so that you discover what works best in supporting you.

Treatments are administered through procedures or infusions given in clinic or hospital settings as a day or in-patient; or through medication often taken at home. Radiotherapy happens in cancer centres in hospital, as a day or in-patient. All the practices can be used anywhere. We might imagine that they will be needed most with the more arduous hospital treatments – and this might be so. However, it might be especially skilful to take your treatment medication at home supported by a practice.

As with the waiting practice, we start with a key Treatment Practice.

Mindful treatment practice

Feet on the Floor (if sitting) or Body on the Bed (if lying) ... *Moving your attention to the contact between the soles of your feet and the floor ... ... or the body and what you are lying on ... ... exploring the quality of this contact and how it feels to you ... ... perhaps moving up close to detailed sensations of the balls of the feet or the back of the body ... ... then noticing the solid of the floor or the bed beneath you ... and expanding to include the whole of your body with what you are lying or sitting on ... . then when you are ready, **Coming to the Breath** as it breathes within the body ... ... Coming up close to the breath, noticing the movement of the breath as it breathes in and as it breathes out ... . at some point, widening to a sense of the breath in the body as a whole and the contact with the floor and the bed supporting you.*

As you follow this practice, with whatever treatment you are having, see if you can open to 'receive' the treatment in a positive way – in your heart as well as into your body. At first, this might feel like a step too far. However, when you are used to the treatment process, and settle into the practice, becoming really familiar with it, (perhaps practicing it at times outside treatment) you may find you can gently begin to affirm, allow and welcome all the potential benefit of the treatment – trusting that you can support yourself with practice to manage the effects of the treatment in the days that follow.

Additional Practices Ideas

 Treatment with kindness

Follow the **Treatment Practice** *of the Feet on the Floor/Body on the Bed and Coming to the Breath ... ... and once you feel settled with this ... ... then looking around at the others having treatment with you, (or near you if they are out of sight) ... ... and internally offering them your* **Kindly Good Wishes** *... ... ... repeating some kindness phrases silently and internally, if you would like to:*

> *'May you be safe in the midst of fear'*
> *'May your treatment be helpful in the midst of your illness'*
> *'May you be peaceful in the midst of anxiety'*

Changing the phrases to suit you ... ... and if it feels alright, including everyone having treatment at this time, wherever they are.

> *'May we all be safe in the midst of fear'*
> *'May all our treatments be helpful in the midst of our illness'*
> *'May we all be peaceful in the midst of anxiety.'*

As before, seeing if it is possible to gently open to the all the potential benefits of your treatment, in your heart, body and mind.

Some of you may have a religious faith, or a personal belief system. You may like to follow practices or prayers that you have used for some time, or used to use some time ago. During treatment, or when waiting, these can nourish and support us. The following practice offers ways of combining mindfulness with your own spiritual practice.

Treatment and blessing

Following the **Treatment Practice** of Feet on the Floor/Body on the Bed and Coming to the Breath ... ... *and once you feel settled with this... ... ... using your own words in the form of a **personal prayer** ... ... Perhaps planning this ahead of treatment by bringing a poem, or a written prayer or phrases that you can repeat to yourself that feel nurturing and helpful... ... ... and/or you might want to bring to mind a special person, real or imaginary, that you feel connected to ... ... Seeing this being as clearly as possible in your mind's eye, and asking for his or her **blessing** ... ... You may want to visualize the chemotherapy, radiotherapy, drug or other treatment, entering you gently in the form of a blessing or maybe as light, love or healing ... ... connecting to the treatment as something that is intended to help and heal you.*

Treatment and visualization

This practice deliberately uses creative visualization. It may be helpful when having radiotherapy, when we are on our own for the short period of the treatment. Some radiotherapy suites have 'light shows' up on the ceiling. You might use these to enhance your visualization.

Following the **Treatment Practice** of Feet on the Floor/ Body on the Bed and Coming to the Breath ... ... *and once you feel reasonably settled into this... ... bring to mind a favourite place in nature... ... ... seeing it in your mind's eye... ... the colours, the shapes ... ... the movements of the trees ... ... the flow of the water perhaps ... the spaciousness of the sky ... ... maybe finding someplace to sit, in your mind's eye ... drinking in all that surrounds you ... ... perhaps feeling the sun gently warming your skin ... ... The wind in your hair ... ... Breathing it all in, as best you can ... ...*

For head and neck radiotherapy

You may need to use a mask to protect your face, if you are having radiotherapy to your head or neck area. Some people find it helps to get creative:

Following the **Treatment Practice** of Feet on the Floor/Body on the Bed and Coming to the Breath ... ... *and once you feel reasonably settled into this ... ... start creating shapes and colours as if you could paint these onto your mask ... ... be specific in your colour schemes ... ... what suits you ? ... ... what might you create it for? A masked ball? An assignation? A disguise?... ... keeping some background awareness of your breath breathing ... ... and continuing to 'craft' your mask over your treatments, changing things as you go – anything goes!*

Juliet followed this practice enthusiastically. She was a talented artist and sculptor and at a party to celebrate the end of her treatment, her radiotherapy mask took pride of place, awash with colour. It was a work of art!

Practice with specific tests and scans

On some occasions, we may need to have scans or tests that require us to stay very still. It may be helpful to bring a favourite longer mindfulness practice with you into the scanner.

When John was in intensive care, his nurse noticed how much more settled he seemed after listening to the Body Scan. A week or so later, he needed to have an MRI scan to assess how he was. He was clearly anxious about keeping still in a contained space, especially as he was having difficulty with his breathing at the time. She suggested that they play that 'recording that you use' into the scanner.

'It wasn't too bad at all', John told me. 'I could keep quite still thanks to the practice. In fact the nurses were so impressed that they asked me to get them a Body Scan CD to play for others.'

Clothing

> Anna always wore her favourite colours when she went for treatment.
> She wore a deep blue blouse for her first chemo. It was a colour that she
> felt good in. People commented on how well she looked. 'It was really
> reassuring', she said. 'After that, I always wore my favourite colours
> whenever I went for treatment.'

Surgery

> Jeremy was very nervous about having surgery. He reflected with his
> partner on what might help. They decided that he would try to make a bit
> of a connection with the staff he came across.
>
> On the day of his surgery, he noticed the porter who wheeled him
> down to theatre. They did not speak much, but Jeremy gained a tangible
> sense of kindness from this man. It was comforting. While waiting out-
> side theatre, a pregnant nurse stood beside his trolley. They got into con-
> versation about her baby and the time passed surprisingly easily. He
> genuinely wished her well when they said goodbye and he was wheeled
> into theatre.
>
> 'It was all so much better than I expected', he said afterwards. 'I
> noticed how kind people were and this definitely helped me feel less
> anxious. Talking to the staff took my mind away from dwelling on what
> was coming next.'

Practicing with the side effects of treatment

If you experience pain or discomfort after surgery or other treatments, your
practice can support you. Rather than tightening around the area, or anticipating
things getting worse – you can practice breathing into it; bringing the breath
around it; feeling the support of the bed or the floor beneath you; and repeating
those kindness phrases to yourself. Be sure to include the pain and the wound
in your kindness phrases – practicing this especially at times when you feel
alone or afraid.

Summary

Remembering your waiting practices. *Coming back*, over and over, to your feet on the floor and the contact of your body with what is supporting you. The feelings of anxiety may not go away, or even change much in intensity, but you are offering them a steadier base. It is a bit like children's jelly served on a paper plate! Disaster is imminent as the jelly easily wobbles off the plate onto the floor. Put it on a bigger and firmer plate, and it has a much better chance of safely staying put, wobbly or no.

Shirley especially liked the good wishes practice. She would repeat the phrases to herself when she was having her infusions in the day unit – offering good wishes to everyone else having treatment around her. It helped her feel more peaceful. She found this a bit curious, but continued anyway. In time, she included the medical staff and then the people down the corridor on the ward, and even the rather odd man in the bed next to her, who kept talking. Little by little, she got into the habit of widening it out to all sorts of people, including her family and friends. 'May we all be safe and well even in the midst of pain and illness', she would say quietly to herself.

Intention For The 'Month' Of Coming Back

Take as long as you need to work through this chapter – doing this in whatever way serves you best. Here are the practices and approaches for you to follow over this next period. All of them are available to download.

Practices – for each 2 week period

Core Practice	– Mindful Walking [10+ times] *Alternating with Body Scan if you choose to*
Short Practices	– Standing in Mountain [ideally daily] – Coming to the Breath [2 or 3 × a day] *Continuing with The Pause and Feet on the Floor*
Exercise	*Reflecting on a pleasant experience every day*

Cancer Practice – with the thread

Waiting Practice	– The Pause & Feet on the Floor (combined)
Treatment practice	– Feet on the Floor & Coming to the Breath (combined)

It may look like a lot. We have been laying down the foundations of a mindfulness-based approach. All that follows later needs to rest on what we establish here, so it is important to ensure that your practice and understanding is well grounded.

Intention

It always helps to reconnect with your intention.

What really matters to you?
How can you bring that into everyday reality?

We are learning that mindfulness has the potential to help us respond more wisely and kindly to the ups and downs of life. So checking that you have reminders in place to help you remember your practices:

- a thread on your wrist
- some coloured sticky dots stuck onto strategic objects
- an app on your phone
- tell others of what you intend
- record your plans in your notebook
- be creative!

You may not manage the practices every single day, but being willing to start over, again and again is a skilful intention. Be sure to appreciate your efforts – day by day, step by step, moment by moment is how we thread mindfulness slowly and surely into our lives.

Notes

1 Frankl, V.E. (1984)
2 Killingsworth, A.M., & Gilbert, D.T. (2010)
3 Macmillan Cancer Support. (2007)
4 Kabat-Zinn, J. (1990, 2013)
5 Suzuki, S. (1973)
6 Rilke, R.M. (1996)
7 Mayne, M. (1995) (Letters written by the then Dean of Westminster to his grandchildren.)
8 Goldstein, J. (2002)
9 If you are using a wheelchair, the same principles apply as in mindful walking. You would bring detailed awareness to the movement of your arms, the contact of your body and any subtle movements of the body that relate to the experience of moving.
10 This exercise follows the same format as that described within MBCT for Depression (Segal, Teasdale and Williams, 2013).
11 The Blob first appeared in Bartley, T. (2012)
12 'Breathing with' was first developed by Jon Kabat-Zinn within MBSR.
13 These kindness phrases used with '*in the midst of*' were first taught me by Christina Feldman and have proved to be very helpful to many people with cancer and others.

Heading Home

Over mountains,
a cloak of rolling clouds
for the noble standing
of the Nantlle kings.

At their feet, the silken surface of lake,
with ripples spread
like drops of kindness from the heart
of the lovely Baladeulyn queen.

And in the wide clear openness above,
a lone circling buzzard –
calling.

We hold freeze-framed these sights and sounds,
a teaching in the body mind.
Etching in us, intent –
to come back.

North Wales (2010)

Nantlle is the name of a dramatic mountain ridge in Snowdonia, North Wales. Lake Baladeulyn lies beneath the Nantlle ridge, in sight of Snowdon, the highest mountain in Wales. Trigonos is the name of the centre in the village of Nantlle and beside the lake, where many mindfulness retreats and workshops are held.

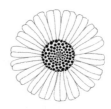

Personal Story

Caroline

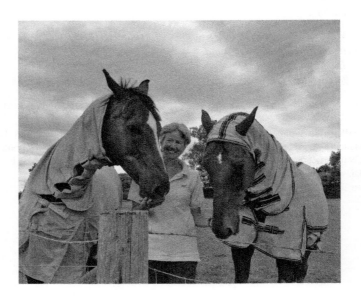

Caroline is 54, married, with two boys in their early 20s. She lives in a rural area and loves the outdoors. She has acquired a horse since having cancer and likes to be physically active. She was first diagnosed with breast cancer two years ago.

Diagnosis

I stopped work the day after my diagnosis. I had surgery within 10 days, and chemotherapy followed that. I went from being fit and well, to living with something I knew I could die from in the near future. I had never been hit by anything even remotely like that and I understood the implications immediately.

I had gone for the biopsy on my own. I assumed you would have to wait for results, and I was amazed to be told that afternoon that – yes I had breast cancer, yes it was malignant, and yes it was already in the lymph nodes. It was even graded that very day. I was told that I needed immediate surgery. So I came home feeling quite numb. This was quickly followed by a sense of horror.

The main horror was having to tell the boys. My older son was at home and I remember J and I sitting and telling him. We were both in tears. He was upset at first, but then seemed to cope with it well. He was soon to go away for some weeks. I didn't want to stop him going, but there was this awful fear that I wouldn't see him again. That was the worst of everything. I care for my mother and my aunt. It was a big issue to tell my mother, who has dementia, and then tell her again and again, because she had forgotten.

There were very few people I felt I could talk to. Most people are initially very shocked and then they keep asking "How are you"? You have had major surgery, followed by chemotherapy and then radiotherapy. So for six months, it is very hard to pretend that everything is fine. I wanted to hide myself away, but the only time I got any semblance of feeling better was outside. So I couldn't hide too much, because I wanted to go for walks, if I physically could.

I'm definitely much more comfortable with it all now, but I don't how I will cope if or when it recurs. I'm aware that it is almost certainly 'when'. The 'if' has become slightly bigger, I suppose and grown into a possibility. I can start to consider a future of some sort – whereas up to now, the future was not somewhere I wanted to go at all. In many ways, mindfulness has helped with that, because it took me away from avoiding planning a future – to focusing on the present.

Treatment

I choose not to remember too much. I found it hard to be physically ill, because I like to be active. My brain felt numb. I couldn't even read a book. I had Herceptin for a year and that also had an effect, but not as bad as chemo. The radiotherapy was worse than I expected. I realized that I didn't have to have it, but I also knew that I would regret not having it if I had a recurrence. I developed a frozen shoulder as a result of radiotherapy and that gave me a lot of problems afterwards.

Psychological impact

I didn't sleep through the night for months and months. I would be awake several times for quite long periods. Physically I was uncomfortable, but mentally I was completely shot. If you are tired all through the day, it makes everything much worse. I felt as if my mind was shut down. I went from being able to read a scientific paper and absorb and retain what I needed with no effort, to sitting staring at the newspaper for hours, without it meaning anything. I think I was traumatized. I didn't think at the time 'this is trauma'. I just thought I needed help. I needed someone to talk to, who could give me an idea of what I was facing and how to come through it.

I was lucky to have a friend who had a similar diagnosis a year before. Seeing her was the first positive thing that happened. She looked and sounded normal, and she smiled. I needed that. Some sort of professional support would have been really helpful, but nothing was offered. Mindfulness wasn't offered. It was only through my friend telling me about it that I connected with it. The medical side of it – the pain and disruption – I could cope with. It was the mental side that was so incredibly difficult.

Confronting mortality is not something that we do. However brave you are, it is a hard thing to come to terms with. I'm not sure if you ever do – but it's something that mindfulness allowed me to think about – later. That was always my main aim in doing mindfulness – to come to a level of acceptance of where I was.

Mindfulness

At the start, I was very sceptical that mindfulness would make any difference. Had it not been for the encouragement of B, my close friend, I would never have done it. I spoke on the phone to the teacher and it made sense to wait until after the chemo had finished. A diagnosis of cancer laid me open to any suggestion. I needed to find ways of moving forward, but at the time, it seemed pretty impossible.

I didn't find it difficult to do the practices. I had the time and I found it quite soothing, almost straight away. It was helpful to be in the group – not something I'd ever done before. You were allowed to opt out, although I didn't feel the need to. I benefitted from seeing where other people were coming from, and how they were coping, and at times struggling. It helped to share ideas and experiences. The whole concept of kindness was not something I'd ever thought of before, not even in my professional training. I found it very helpful.

About five/six weeks into the course, I was outside gardening – it was a spring day – and I had this sudden realization that I was comfortable, mentally. I had been digging and I stopped and I could hear the birds sing. I could see the leaves starting – and I was suddenly at one again. I attributed this directly to mindfulness. I felt content – comfortable with the situation. I had not felt like that for a long time and certainly not since the diagnosis. It felt naturally good. It was a bit deeper than mood, which comes and goes. There was this realization that I was content. I will occasionally get moments like that now, and I recognize them more and more.

Mindfulness practice now

I come and go with it. I don't do a formal practice for weeks on end, and then I might come back to it regularly for a week. I don't think it is associated with times of stress but perhaps it is. I find the Body Scan most relaxing. I rarely get through it without falling asleep, but I always wake up before the end and feel great. And that is not to do with falling asleep, because I can have a snooze during the day and when I wake I don't feel anything like the same as when I've done a Body Scan.

I am aware of mindfulness quite frequently during the day. It is not always deliberate – but I often just stop, especially when I'm outside – and that is a little practice. Yesterday I was filling the manure bags and the chickens chose to come round me and they were pecking away – and I stopped to watch them. But it was not just watching - it was bigger than that – I was aware. I was content.

When I have a distressing situation, like waiting at the doctors', I will often come to the breath. I find that helps. So I use bits of it frequently, but I haven't pursued it as much as I thought I would, when the course finished.

What has getting cancer offered you?

After I stopped work there was a certain relief. It has been one of the odd positive aspects about the whole situation – I have been given time to reflect – time for myself - and the chance to have a horse, which I've always wanted.

These two years have offered me an opportunity to think about lots of deeper issues. Why are we here? What are we doing? What do we leave behind? What do I want to achieve in the time I have left?

It has offered me a certain freedom to live for the moment and not worry about the future. In a physical sense, it has given me the spur to get on and do things now, because I don't know where I will be in six months. It has changed my priorities. It may have made J and I stronger. It has made us talk about things and made me realize how much he would do for me. I think I am more content with my life now than I was before.

Whether it is getting cancer, or no longer working, or whether it is mindfulness – I don't know. It is probably a combination of all sorts of things that has meant that I'm happier now than I've been for a long time. And I think I'm more able to face whatever comes next. I'm more aware of what makes me happy and of the things that aren't important. I have found it hard to continue friendships with some of the people who I was close to before. My priorities have changed.

Many things are a lot less significant. I am very grateful for this time – although I don't know to whom. My boys are my great priorities. They are getting older and more able to cope with life. It must be so devastating for people who get cancer and have young families. It fills me with great sadness thinking about that.

The future is still frightening, but I don't dwell on it. I feel at a bit of a crossroads now – what do I want to achieve? What do I want to do with my life? I've lived for two years since being diagnosed, but that is no guarantee. I am physically much better. I have this need to give back and yet I'm not quite sure how or why or where. I don't think that I resent cancer any more – and I certainly did to start with. I am lucky to have had this time and I am grateful for the support I have had.

The Journey

I walk the path more softly now.
I pause, I feel, I think.
Yet, still, sometimes, I sink
into the abyss that is the future,
or the past.

But now we hear the birdsong, above the ticking clock.
We stretch up to the mountain, together and alone,
and wait
for the sunrise of compassion to peep across the summit
and bathe the starfish held gently in our hands.

In silence, I stare into the cool lake.
I see the blue sky behind the darkening thoughts
as I search for the anchor within
to bring me to my peace,
and home.

Caroline

Chapter 3

Turning Towards

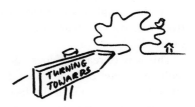

What happens to you, uncontrollable or otherwise, isn't the important thing. What matters is simply how you are with it. And you can always, always, choose that. Knowing this provides meaning and purpose even amidst great pain and sadness.

Kate Gross[1]

Turning Towards is our third movement. It proposes a radically different and essentially gentle way of relating to suffering.

We start by exploring our natural tendency to turn away from what troubles us and learn a range of ways of responding, depending on the strength of the difficulty. There are some new key practices and we review the ones you have been practicing. In the experience of cancer section, we move to the period immediately after treatment. This is often a time of intense anxiety. We share some practices dedicated to managing uncertainty.

As we develop these new skills and approaches, it is vital that we stay connected to Intention and Coming Back. Each new movement rests on the ones before.

Intention supports us to:

- Remain true to what really matters.
- Remember and reconnect with this

   Coming Back helps us to:

- Bring attention to present moment experience.
- Notice when the mind wanders off and come back.

Mindfulness: A Kindly Approach to Being with Cancer, First Edition. Trish Bartley.
© 2017 John Wiley & Sons, Ltd. Published 2017 by John Wiley & Sons, Ltd.
Companion Website: www.wiley.com/go/bartley/mindfulness

Turning Away – A Natural Reaction

We all try to avoid unpleasant experiences. This seems perfectly obvious. Even the simplest of organisms instinctively pull back and move away from whatever obstructs or threatens them. Their very survival often relies on it.

This way of reacting does not serve us well – yet we are hardwired to deal with stress and difficulty like this. It helped our forager ancestors in their attempts to stay safe in the face of dangerous sabre tooth tigers – and it is obviously lifesaving when we need to react quickly, such as when a toddler runs into traffic. However, events like a missed train connection or having a difficult exchange may well trigger this same threat response.

The human nervous system cannot easily tell the difference between a range of difficult experiences. It reacts by always being on the lookout for threat. Most everyday situations, stressful as they might be, need a more skilful and nuanced response. They cannot be settled in a moment. Running away or having an argument does not help – in fact often makes things worse. Yet this is how we are instinctively drawn to act.

Recognizing aversion

When a number of significant stressors combine, we struggle to manage. The mind, in attempting to fix things, moves automatically into flight/fight mode, instinctively activating a threat response. Unpleasant experiences (e.g. having a very long wait in clinic) become stressful and potentially overwhelming when fuelled by judgement and potential scenarios ('I can't manage another minute more' and/or 'How come everyone else looks so calm?' and 'What is wrong with me?').

Things we may have managed reasonably well before diagnosis, may now loom large and have much more impact. We fall into old patterns, perhaps becoming withdrawn, tense and irritable. Sleep gets tricky, anxiety increases and mood goes down. Stress hormones release affecting the digestive and immune system, and increasing the heart rate. Aches and pains appear in the body as a result of all the tension. This last is a particularly distressing symptom for anyone who has had a cancer diagnosis – as it is often interpreted catastrophically as a sign of recurrence.

If patterns of stress happen now and then, we manage reasonably well, weathering the storms when they hit. However, when the challenges build, one thing crowding in on the next, we suffer greatly and can feel overwhelmed.

The tendency to add extra

Let us look at this pattern a little closer.

Our reactivity to difficulty and stress is often influenced by ancient patterns that trigger stress reactivity. First, difficulty arises and then, our reactions follow. The difficulty is often unavoidable. All sorts of things happen that we have little or no control over. Whilst we may not be able to influence the difficulty, we *can* change is our reaction. This is exactly what we are learning in relation to mindfulness – to *choose our response* to what we find difficult, in ways that are supportive and helpful – rather than *reacting* in knee-jerk and instinctive ways that often add extra on top of what is already there.

Birth, old age, sickness and death

Being diagnosed with cancer is a significant life event. Rationally of course, we all know that we can get sick and that one day we will die. Yet we act as if illness and death happen to everyone else. Having to face your own mortality *is* shocking. It does not seem to matter what age you are. I have met people in their 80s, who are shattered at getting a diagnosis of cancer.

Once treatment has finished, we imagine we will resume our 'normal' lives – yet the reality of having a life threatening illness changes one's view of life profoundly. 'I too will die one day – maybe sooner than I thought' – is now a present reality. It is hard to process this.

Tigers above, tigers below

There is a very old mythical story[2] of someone running from tigers:

> *She runs and runs until she comes to a cliff. Seeing no other way to escape, she climbs down and hangs on to a little plant. Then she sees there are tigers below her as well. When she looks more carefully at what she is holding onto, she sees a mouse gnawing away at the roots. She looks up – tigers above. She looks down – tigers below. She looks at the mouse – and then she notices a little clump of strawberries growing beside her. She picks one, places it in her mouth, and eats it mindfully. It is delicious!*

I love this story. It is quite ridiculous and rather wonderful. The woman in the story tries to run from the tigers, but is unable to get free of them. They keep on coming. Fighting the tigers was never an option. So what is she to do? She stops and eats a strawberry!

What does it mean? Tigers above and tigers below is often interpreted as a metaphor for birth and death. We cannot escape either and they chase us from the very beginning to the very end of our lives. Both involve pain, fear and suffering. Both hold uncertainty – for we never know when the actual moment of birth or death will happen, or what it will bring. Inevitably we try to avoid, deny and resist what threatens life and brings us up close to our mortality.

How to manage the distress and uncertainty and live as fully as possible? How to notice and enjoy the strawberry?

Just as the tigers chasing are symbolic of birth, old age, illness and death hounding us until the very end, so the strawberry is surely a metaphor for being awake, alive and present to what is precious.

Daniel was in his mid-40s, when he was diagnosed with cancer. He had meditated off and on since being a teenager and started again by practicing mindfulness, when introduced to it a few months before his diagnosis.

Nature and creativity held great significance for him. One of his favourite practices was 'Standing in Mountain' – or sitting imagining the abiding presence of mountain within his body. It offered him a strong sense of feeling grounded, stable and present. He had grown up in Iceland, and often talked fondly of the country's volcanoes and mud pools.

When he contracted pneumonia, we developed a practice in which Daniel imagined he had shoes made of lava. He could breathe up through the imaginary air bubbles under his feet and stay calm. Instead of feeling panic, fearing not being able to breathe, he could connect with his beloved country and find his breath in amongst the volcanoes, steam and the lava at his feet.

Let us draw together what we have explored so far – and then continue by discovering how we can relate differently to what we find difficult.

Summary

We have a natural fight/flight instinct towards the unwanted and the difficult.

Distress is triggered by the tendency of the mind to judge, blame, move into catastrophe, and compare (see Chapter 2 and the tendencies of mind).

These tendencies add 'extra' on top of unavoidable unpleasant or difficult experiences. Reactivity creates and intensifies our suffering.

It is therefore important that we find ways of relating differently to unavoidable difficulties without making them bigger. This involves us in learning to respond by cultivating new habits of mind.

Relating Kindly To The Difficult

Care, balance and stability is needed when responding to difficulty. We learn that when we relate kindly to challenging experience the grip of suffering loosens.

Choosing how to respond

As the practice of Coming Back gets established, we learn to spot the signs of upcoming 'weather'. A judging inner commentary, a difficult storyline, a dip in mood, or a familiar clench in the belly, are all pointers that something challenging has arrived. Noticing these 'warning signs' is the first step to mindfully responding.

If we do nothing, and fail to notice and acknowledge that difficulty is brewing, we are likely to react with habitual patterns of avoiding, or even pushing away the difficulty. This reactivity is what triggers our suffering.

Instead, on a good day, we remember to:

- Stop and **Pause to Notice** what is going on (body, thoughts, emotions, storyline, etc.).
- Bring attention to **Feet on the Floor** and **Coming to the Breath** (coming back to the anchor of the present moment) and stepping out of automatic pilot.
- We then **Gauge the Intensity** of what we are experiencing, and
- **Choose** a **response** wisely.

We have two immediate alternatives:

A If the unpleasant experience is mild to moderate – we can choose *Turning Towards The Difficulty*, exploring a felt sense of it in the body.
B However, if there is a rapid build of intensity and a risk of feeling overwhelmed, then we wisely make the choice of *Finding Another Place to Stand*.

A Turning Towards The Difficulty – *mild to moderate challenge*[3]

1 Noticing the felt sense of difficulty in the body

The body is a bit like a barometer that alerts us to change in our 'emotional' weather. Any experience, thought or emotion makes itself felt in the body. So whenever something unpleasant or difficult arises, there will always be a resonance within the body – a felt sense of that difficulty. Increasingly, we learn to notice and relate to this.

2 Exploring the physical sensations involved

Where can I feel the sensation?
Look in the trunk of the body. This is where sensitive feelings make themselves felt.
What is the shape of the sensation?
Is it round? Does it have edges?
Does it have colour, texture, weight, temperature or movement?
We are sculpting the sensation – just like an artist might – being creative and curious, noticing any changes in intensity, size or shape as we do.

3 Breathing into the sensations

Just as you did in the Body Scan when you found tender places – bringing the breath into the body as if it were gently flowing around the felt sense of difficulty in the trunk of the body.

4 Bringing kindness in on the breath

Imagining that kindness could flow in on the breath, touching the sensations of difficulty in the body – like a warm breeze on a cool day. Letting the breath be the vehicle for kindness.

Some things to remember

We are not trying to get rid of the difficulty – counter intuitive, as this may seem. The practice is to hold the difficulty in awareness – gently and with curiosity. This is our primary intention. We do this by exploring the sensations in the body, rather than getting into the stories in the mind. A tendency to ruminate gets us stuck in repetitive loops of thinking and inner commentary. These simply dig us deeper.

Physical sensations have a different quality to thoughts or emotions. They are slower and do not change so quickly. We learn to be curious about them – coming to read and rely on these body messages to see what is present.

We build this practice gradually – this is important - starting with something straightforward. Just like an athlete learning her skill on the high jump, we slowly increase the height of the bar as we gain confidence, courage and practice experience.

Sitting on a park bench

When experiencing a persistent difficulty that feels hard to be with, I sometimes imagine that I am sitting on a park bench beside it. There are lots of different sizes of benches – two person benches, and some much bigger ones that could seat as many as eight to 10 people. Depending on the difficulty, I decide which imaginary bench size I might choose to sit on. I do not look across at my difficult 'companion' or start a conversation. I just imagine that I am sitting on the bench with as much space as I want, between us. Noticing how this feels and breathing with it.

Going towards the neutral

A woman in a mindfulness class was struggling to get in touch with her physical sensations. Everything in the body felt miserable, painful, and unwanted. When asked by the teacher if there was anywhere that felt okay – she replied by saying that her left big toe was quite 'happy'. This was a revelation to her. She learned to turn to her big toe when something was difficult.

Sometimes choosing to pay attention to something neutral or mundane is just what we need to do. When James was introduced to mindfulness, there was no raisin to hand, so he and his teacher used an apple instead. To his surprise, James found it quite calming to hold the apple and pass it from one hand to the other. He sometimes 'practices' with an apple when he is feeling a bit stressed.

Turning Towards takes courage, practice and confidence. We cultivate baby steps at first – not barging through into too much, but not pushing away either.

B Finding Another Place To Stand – strong to intense challenge

There are bound to be times when we are caught unawares. A surge of anxiety comes out of the blue – or painfully difficult thoughts invade the mind. Janice described this like 'a firework rocket going up into the sky.'

Managing the flood

Let us look at how we might manage strong challenges through the metaphor of a flood.

There is a beautiful place[4] near where I live where we hold mindfulness retreats. A small river flows through the grounds. A year or so ago, the river flooded. There had been a lot of rain, but the banks usually manage the water volume pretty well. On this particular day, very few people were around, and the river broke its banks and flooded the car park, the office, the gallery with its beautiful pine floor, and even found its way into the main house.

Afterwards, measures were put in place to reduce the chance of this happening again. The banks were strengthened. The car park was repaired. The office thankfully dried out and the gallery was given an even more beautiful oak floor. In the end, no lasting damage was done, and the river has not flooded since.

What can we learn about flooding?

When conditions conspire, intensity and overwhelm (our version of flooding) can happen. There is no cause for shame, or judgement. If pressure builds and the challenge is considerable, it is natural to feel the impact. What matters is how to support yourself and recover.

When 'flooding'[5] is imminent, we need to move to dry land until the levels subside. Instead of flooding, it might feel as if thick fog is closing in on you, in which case you need to find a safe place to shelter.

With either of these examples, the skill seems to be in:

- noticing the risk of 'flooding'
- making a choice to find another place to stand
- moving to stand there.

This is not a time to turn towards the experience. Instead, we engage our attention somewhere else – whilst the floodwaters recede, or the fog lifts.

There are a number of possible approaches – choosing what works best for you.

1 Moving to be physical

Taking exercise definitely helps us manage intensity. It is why the mindful movement practices are often favourites in MBSR and MBCT courses. They offer a clear alternative focus to engage with.

Depending on your health and fitness levels, some activities may be more appropriate than others. Choosing one to suit you, or finding your own.

Here are some ideas:

- going for a strenuous walk (especially if the weather is wild)
- watching a football match in the open air
- playing some sport
- having a shower or going for a swim
- digging the garden
- engaging in some DIY
- clearing out that cupboard you have been meaning to do for ages (and be sure to admire your efforts afterwards)
- cleaning the house or washing the car (ditto above).

Be vigilant of the mind's tendency to sneak back in and ruminate around what has happened. Keep coming back to your physical sensory experience as best you can.

2 Engaging the senses

Or you can also choose to do something quite different – a new place, a new activity, a new focus of attention.

Nature is a great ally in these situations. We can set the intention to walk attentively, exploring the details of trees or plants around us – or cultivating an open focus to appreciate the space of the sky and the views. People often find it comforting to be outside in natural places – or even to be walking down a street. Our moments of 'flood risk' can be placed on a larger canvas, helping us to realize that they are just that – moments, which shift and change like the landscape and the weather.

Wherever we live, whether in a city or in the countryside, there is always a park to explore, a hill to climb, a beach to walk along, or some gardens to look at. Being outside amongst others can help you to remember that they too have tough times, just like you.

Other options might include:

- visiting an open air market
- going to an art gallery, museum or exhibition

- spending time outside with kind and interesting people
- seeing an uplifting movie.

You may not feel like getting up and going out – but better to make the effort than be overwhelmed and miserable. Find someone to join you – explaining that your intention is to focus on what is engaging and interesting. Retelling the story of your distress will not help just now, however tempting this might be.

Someone who was managing intense emotion wrote about his experience like this:

> At some stage, I stood next to one of the enormous big trees and looked over the valley while emotions were rolling in. I felt very grounded with the help of the tree and very spacious with the help of the valley. It was as if I was giving the emotions this space and groundedness – allowing me to feel them without being washed away by them, and turning towards them eventually with curiosity and wanting to learn from them.

Practice being mindful and aware of what you are doing as you do it. You are not running away. After an afternoon spent in nature, or at an art gallery – even after having a shower, things will have shifted. Nothing stays the same for very long. The intensity may return, but you will be better prepared to respond to it.

After the flood

When things have eased, it would be skilful to gently turn towards the body and see how it is now.

Sitting in an upright chair, or lying on a bed or on the floor, and engaging in a brief, kindly, self-guided body scan (or using the recorded practice).

> *What do you notice in the trunk of the body?*
> *Are there any residual sensations that resonate with the intensity that you felt?*
> *Can you explore them with gently curiosity – breathing into them and bringing kindness in on the breath?*
> *No need to move back into the story of the intensity – but just staying gently in the body and paying kindly attention to what is there.*

Planning ahead for difficult times

Just as it was important to strengthen the riverbanks after the flood, it is wise for us to plan ahead when intense difficulty is likely.

What are the situations that you find especially difficult?
What might be the most helpful response?
How can you prepare for this?

Perhaps choosing to record these triggers and tendencies in your note-book – including the strategies and plans that you might put in place to respond to them. Writing them down helps us to remember, especially when feelings are strong.

Summary of relating kindly to difficulty

- We spot the difficult feelings as they are building – remembering that if we do nothing, we will react automatically by tightening and avoiding (which adds extra).
- We **Pause To Notice** and **Gauge The Intensity** of the experience; and **Choose a response** wisely.
- If the difficulty is manageable (mild to moderate), we practice **Turning Towards the Difficulty** – by noticing the felt sense in the body; exploring the sensations; breathing into them; and bringing kindness in on the breath.
- If the difficulty is intense, we practice **Finding Another Place To Stand** – by getting physically active; or by engaging the senses in nature, or through some interesting activity.

A third option, which we now explore is Turning Towards the Lovely as an alternative way of responding to all levels of difficulty.

Turning Towards The Lovely

A radical way of responding

Experience shows that the mind inclines itself towards whatever it habitually dwells on. If we repeatedly worry about the future – or often fantasize negative scenarios – the mind tends to slip into these places more readily. This will fuel anxiety and may become an established pattern of mind.

Turning Towards what is lovely is a way of countering this slide into negative automatic habits of mind. It is not remotely the same as 'positive thinking'.

We are not denying what is difficult – nor making things artificially positive.

We are simply choosing to place attention on what we love and enjoy, instead of dwelling on what is difficult. In the fog of our minds, and the busyness of our lives, we may be unaware when the sun has come out or notice the sparkles of light amongst the trees from the rain that fell last night. It is always up to us to notice what is there. Will you feed what is painful by dwelling on your worst fears? Or can you grow the capacity to appreciate what you delight in, even in the midst of difficult times?

Ordinary happiness comes and goes. It is here one minute with a piece of chocolate cake and gone the next when the moment has passed, or the mood has changed. Appreciation and even contentment emerges more from within. They connect with what has meaning for us and where we place our focus.

> *If someone had seen our faces on the journey from Auschwitz to a Bavarian camp, as we beheld the mountains of Salzburg with their summits glowing in the sunset, through the little barred windows of the prison carriage, he would never have believed that those were the faces of men who had given up all hope of life and liberty ... {yet} we were carried away by nature's beauty.*[6]

Gladdening the mind

When we reflect on all the unknown people who have made our lives possible, we realize there are countless numbers that we are indebted to. There is a Sri Lankan saying, 'I delight you are here'.[7] You can experiment with this. When feeling a bit flat, I sometimes practice this at the foot of two silver birch trees, which my son and I planted many years ago.

The Navajo Indians[2] teach their children to appreciate the sun. When they are old enough, they take them out at dawn to watch the sun rising up out of the horizon. They tell the children that the sun will only live for one day, so it is important that they do not waste the day.

Others like me

Turning Towards what we appreciate links us directly with others, in our awareness of what they too experience. They are people who have joys and sorrows like me – who get ill, who get well, like me.

There are places and people that bless us with their beauty and love. This can show itself in many different ways. My daughter and I can be overcome with laughter, tears pouring down our faces. It is precious beyond words. Generous giving and kindness can greatly nourish us. Joy wakes us up to what is well in us – what is free from pain – what is whole.

In conclusion

Here is a story that illustrates what we have been exploring.

Some years ago, a group of Western trekkers were walking through a dramatic Himalayan valley. The route went along the bottom of an almost dry Kali Gandaki river, through a canyon, said to be the deepest in the world. A strong wind blew up the gorge, pelting grey grit from the riverbed directly into their faces. Wrapped up from head to toe, they could just about make out the track ahead. Head down, one foot in front of the other, it took immense effort to make it through.

On the way back, they took a different route. This time higher, at one side of the gorge, it was possible to look down and see the monotone grey of the valley floor below, and remember that long walk, and that unkind wind. What struck them powerfully was the astonishing beauty of the place from this different perspective. Rising up from the ground were sheer cliffs of pale granite rock – with houses somehow built into them – and a few pine trees somehow growing out of them. Further up were thicker layers of dark green and then the snow line. At the top was the summit of the magnificent Dhaulagiri, the seventh highest mountain in the world. It was adorned with a crisp snow peak – above which was the glorious deep blue of the sky. It was necessary to bend the head back to see all this – so vast was the scope from the top to the bottom. It was an extraordinary sight – one that they had entirely failed to appreciate when they first walked into the place.

The message of the landscape seems clear. Head down, we are buffeted by the dramas of life. We fail to look up and appreciate what is around us. Closed in by the claustrophobia of suffering, we feel quite alone – yet invariably there are others, just like me going through something similar.

A different view, a new perspective offers an opportunity to appreciate and connect. This opens our understanding and enables us to cultivate a different relationship to the things that challenge us most.

The Thickening Stillness

Silence rolls in like mist
across the shores of our short history
boundaries erected in haste
cease to be.

A pause, a glimpse, a heartbeat
leap out, then fade away
breath slowing, deepening
sighing release.

An inscape revisited
a nakedness re-touched
and in the depth of the fire
and in the depth of the earth
only this:
compassion
and clear light.

"But you said ..." and "she said ..."
"and you did" and "he did"
fading and retreating
and in the thickening stillness
healing begins.

Stewart Mercer (2002)

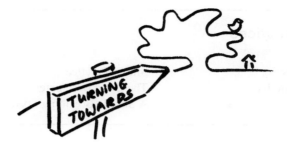

The Practices, A Model, And Some Exercises

Allowing difficult feelings, thoughts, sensations and inner experiences means that we willingly let them remain in awareness, without demanding that they change or be other than they are.[8]

Overview

We look at some new key practices – a core practice and two short ones. We review the previous chapter's practices and explore some new exercises, a cognitive model and some ways of recognizing your personal patterns.

Review thus far

Moving on now to ask:

Am I ready to cultivate mindfulness practice in a more radical, confident and courageous way?
Is my practice sufficiently established to move to a deeper level?

Is it familiar for you to doubt your next steps? Maybe you can reflect on this internally, perhaps walking with it – and see what is best. Trusting your own answers.

New Practices

Core practice	– Sitting Practice
Short Practices	– The Body Barometer
	– A Simple Breathing Space

Core Practice

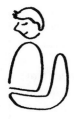

Sitting Practice

Finding a place to sit. Perhaps choosing a straight back chair and planting your feet flat on the floor, sitting slightly away from the back of the chair, if that is comfortable for you. You can support your back with a cushion at the bottom of the spine, if that feels best. Sitting tall, relaxed and comfortable, as best you can. Or you may have a stool or meditation cushion that you prefer to use. Ensure that your hips are higher than your knees, which are well supported.

There are a number of sections in the sitting practice. Include sections 1 and 2 every time at the start – and then choose others to follow.

---

1 Sitting Practice – taking your seat and connecting with intention

Taking your seat by turning attention to the base of the body and its connection with the floor and with whatever you're sitting on … … Feeling the points of contact … the weight of the body moving down, held by the floor … … Now when you're ready, including a sense of the height of the body moving up … … the spine lifting up out of the pelvis, up through the back … shoulders balancing either side of the spine … … chin slightly tucked, feeling that little stretch up the back of the neck … and then extending up through the middle of the head, to the top of the back of the crown of the head … …

Sitting tall, grounded, present … dignified … … with the possibility of strong back … … and soft front … …

When you are ready, coming to your intention for this practice … … remembering that the deepest intention lies in the heart … … so including kindliness for yourself and all that matters to you.

2 Coming to the Breath

Turning your attention now to become aware of the breath … … as it moves in the body … … … Where do you feel the breath most vividly? … … … … … is it in the chest? … or perhaps the belly? … or maybe some

---

place in between the two … … … choosing for yourself where you will rest your attention to experience the breath in all its fullness … … … … … from the very beginning to the very end ….

If at any point, you notice that the mind has wandered, remember that this is not a problem. It is simply what minds do … … Our task is just to notice, and then patiently and kindly coming back to the breath wherever you find it … … ….

Can you be there at the very moment that the breath starts to breathe in? … … how does that feel to you? … … … … … breathing as if for the first time

'Breath, breathing in, I know I am breathing in'….
'Breath, breathing out, I know I am breathing out'….

3   Expanding into the body as a whole

Now, expanding the attention to include a sense of the body as a whole sitting here … … … … … From the very base to the very top of the body … … from the back to the front … … the full capacity of the body sitting here … … … … … not so much thinking the body, but sensing it directly as it sits here.

And as you do this, you will notice that the breath is still here moving within the body … … … the whole body is breathing … … … … Every cell, every muscle, every part of the body breathing … … … Breathing body.

4   Mindfulness of hearing

Now, we move to become aware of sound … … Expanding the attention further, beyond the body, into the space around you … … … Opening up to receiving sound into the ears … … No need to hunt for it, just letting sounds come to you in the space of your awareness … … … … sound coming and going … … … rising and fading … … perhaps noticing the rhythm, the texture, volume, and quality of sound … … perhaps liking some sounds more than others … …

And if you notice that you are creating stories around the sound, or getting engaged in what is making the sound … … Just knowing that your mind has wondered off into thinking, and that this is not a problem … … Simply coming back to your moment by moment experience of hearing sound, arising out of silence … and coming and going.

5   Present with thinking and feeling

Up to this point, we have related to thoughts as distractions in the mind. Now, we turn to thoughts and feelings as the objects of our awareness ... ... Knowing that at any point, if you get lost, you can always return to the anchor of the breath, breathing deep in the body ... ... For now, opening into a sense of spacious awareness, to become aware of thoughts and feelings as they come and go ... ...

It is as if the mind is like the blue of the sky, vast, clear and spacious ... ... And thoughts and feelings, when they arise, are like weather patterns passing across the sky ... ... Sometimes, the sky of mind is clear and spacious ... ... And then at other times, thoughts arise perhaps accompanied by feelings ... ... No need to get involved with the content of the thought, or the quality of the feeling, but simply noticing how they come and go, sometimes lingering, sometimes more demanding of your attention, ... but however they appear to you, they are simply events in the mind ... ... much like sounds in the space around you, coming and going.

At any time, if you notice that you've become involved with the thought or the feeling, knowing you can always come back to the anchor of the breath ... ...

Choiceless awareness

Finally, practicing with whatever predominates in the mind ... ... So if the breath is centre stage, then mindful of breathing ... ... If sounds show up, being aware of sounds and hearing, ... If sensations in the body come forefront in your experience, then being with them ... And if thoughts or feelings become apparent, just holding them in your awareness, in the sky of mind ... ... being with whatever is there moment by moment ... ...

Knowing that whenever the mind is no longer aware of present experience, but has wandered off somewhere else, it is always possible to come back kindly, to the anchor of the breath, breathing itself deep in the body.

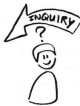

Reflective inquiry

What have you noticed about your experience of the Sitting Practice?
How has that been for you?
What do you make of that, if anything?

Turning to reflective inquiry after each Sitting Practice using the questions as before – or choosing to be more creative, if you like – and developing your own questions. It is incredibly important to continue to reflect on your practice. Without this, it is all too easy for mindfulness to become dull and formulaic. Seeding curiosity into those moments after our practice. 'How was that'? 'What was the quality of my mind'? Not so much judging – 'I practiced well/not well' – but 'what was I cultivating during that practice'?

As with other core practices, you are invited to follow the sitting practice most days, or at least five times a week, for several weeks. These longer core practices enable us to build the momentum of mindfulness, deepening and maturing our skills in practice – and helpful in weaving mindfulness into our lives.

Sitting practice is central to mindfulness and includes many different objects of attention. Some of these, such as awareness of thoughts and feelings, are complex practices in their own right and take time and patience to develop.

Unpleasant Experience

In the last chapter, we looked at Pleasant Experience, using The Blob to map each experience (we will review this a little later in this chapter). We do the same again here – this time choosing to notice unpleasant experiences using the Blob once more to map the different layers. Here is an example to get you started:

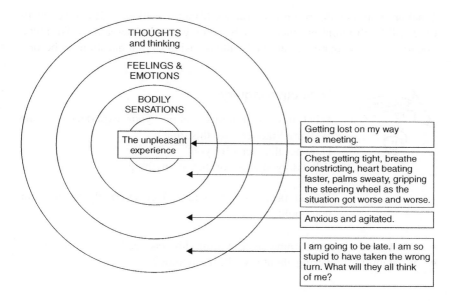

You might feel some resistance to look at something unpleasant, but it offers us valuable learning. There is no need to choose extremely unpleasant experiences. Everyday difficulties will be more useful. They will help you to tease out the different layers of unpleasant experience and discover the patterns within them. An important first step is to bring them into awareness. This exercise helps you learn to do that.

We draw out the learning in the next chapter. For now, see if it is possible to be curious about your unpleasant experiences – in the service of learning, insight and kindly response. Find one every day to investigate.

Home Practice Review

We now reflect on the practices that you have been following from the Coming Back chapter.

Mindful walking practice

What are you noticing when you practice Mindful Walking? Of course, every time will be different but there may be some general observations. We invite you to reflect on your experience of walking, using similar questions as before.

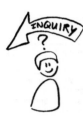

Reflective inquiry

What have you noticed about your experience of the Walking Practice over this time?
How has that been for you?
What do you make of that, if anything?

If you prefer – you can reflect internally or in your notebook:

- What is new in my learning since starting this practice?
- What am I discovering about myself, if anything?

Short Practices

1   Standing In Mountain
2   Coming to the Breath

You are encouraged to continue to review the short and everyday practices you have been following. Can you generate your own questions to help you draw out what you are noticing? Or adapt those that we have used. There is real value in reviewing and reflecting on your practice. It enables your learning to emerge and allows you to bring this into the service of your well-being.

Short reflective inquiry

We are fostering a way of reflecting on the experience of practice *as* and immediately *after* we experience it. This does not require analysis or a deliberately thinking *about* the practice. Instead we are developing *a sense of questioning* about it. This is an important part of mindfulness learning. It does not need to take long. It is more about bringing an attitude of curiosity to your experience – not directed towards 'getting it right' or achieving a 'result' – but in order to genuinely explore what is there, and what learning you can draw from this.

These are the questions we have been using – bringing an orientation of curiosity to your experience.

What did you notice about some aspect of the experience of that practice – in general/in detail?
How was that for you?
What do you make of that, if anything?

Pleasant Experience Exercise

You were invited to pay special attention to your pleasant experiences over the last month – using 'the Blob' to map them.

What did you discover?
What did it take to simply enjoy the (pleasant) moment?

Here is a story from someone who was exploring this exercise:

Tessa had some special friends who had supported her loyally. She had been ill for some years with ovarian cancer and had endured many different treatments. She was no longer able to get out much. 'Whenever we get together, we laugh and laugh', she told me, on one our phone sessions. 'I really value that sense of the ridiculous that we share. The other day, one of them sent me the most stunning roses I have ever seen. I have been just sitting and drinking them in. I can feel all my senses heightened and my heart almost glow – just looking at them, remembering the kindness of my friends.'

Here is another example of a pleasant experience – this time mapped onto a Blob.

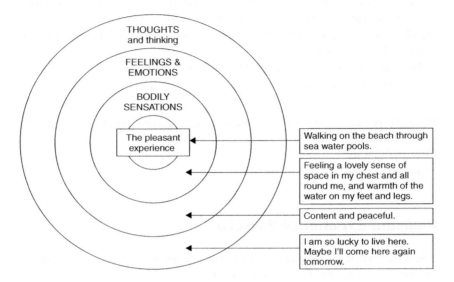

Sometimes, it may have seemed difficult to find anything pleasant to reflect on. Other days there may be many opportunities. Remembering that our pleasant moments can be quite subtle. They do not have to be dramatically wonderful. We are simply learning to notice what is here that we can turn to and enjoy.

It is also not unusual to find some sadness mixed up in the experience of the pleasant. We enjoy a moment's connection and then feel unhappy that it has finished – or we move into thinking that it may never happen quite like that again. See if you can find ways of noticing when thoughts take you away from the present moment and move you to a future anticipated projection. Noticing what is happening and practice Coming Back to how things are right now (pleasant and unpleasant – happy and sad – or however it might be).

Recognizing Our Personal Patterns

We now outline a number of different ways that you can build an understanding of your patterns of reactivity.

The Sea Of Reactions (Part One)

An Exercise

This might be a good process to ask a friend to do with you.

Materials:
- Plenty of A4 plain paper (scrap paper is fine with one side blank)
- Thick marker pen

1   One word reactions

Bring to mind some familiar stressful situations and write one word on a piece of paper in big writing for each of your likely reactions. These might be feelings (e.g. anxious, irritable, etc.) or reactive behaviours (things you do – e.g. watch television, get busy, rush, etc.). *Write one or two words on each piece of paper* – and stick to unhelpful reactions for now. This is not a time to generate helpful ideas! Continue until you cannot think of any more.

Put the sheets of paper (words up) on the floor as each one is written – then stand up and wander around the words, having a good look at them.

Choose one word that you feel drawn to explore a bit more. It might be one that you know is especially unhelpful and typical of how you often react.

2   Exploring the felt sense in the body

Sit down with the word/s you have chosen – and explore where you feel this in the body. If you are doing this with a friend, take it in turns to describe the sensations in the trunk of the body when you react like this (they will have chosen their own word from the floor). Help your partner get right into the detail of these sensations – taking care not to get side-tracked into the story – and simply staying with the felt sense of it in the body. And then you swap over, with your partner helping you - or *vice versa*.

Some words others have written in the Sea of Reactions

blaming	ignoring	frozen	overwhelmed	weeping
angry	trapped	drink	anxious	inadequate
scared	numb	driven	frightened	distraught
alone	brooding	jittery	avoid	frustrated
busy	withdraw	rush	worry	fear the worst
stress	sick	pain	tiny	panic
eat chocolate	tearful	irritated	terror	anticipate
paranoid	guilty	worthless	denial	pick a fight
restless	agitated	can't sleep	annoyed	escape
depressed	resentful	silent	cry	hopeless

At the end of this, reflect on your own or with your friend, on what you have learned. Perhaps turning to a favourite short practice – such as Feet on the Floor and Coming to the Breath – to ensure you are grounded and well connected to the present moment.

Knowing your patterns enables you to recognize the automatic ways you react. You are not on your own here. We all have times when 'our buttons get pressed'. Once you are aware of your own patterns, you are better able to choose a different response. Often, however, we do not recognize the pattern until after the reaction has been played out–but over time, we catch things earlier.

A Vicious Circle Of Anxious Preoccupation[9]

In the service of learning to recognize your patterns, we now look at a psychological model that speaks to the way that many of us react. It outlines a pattern that we can easily fall into, and shows how distress is triggered and can intensify.

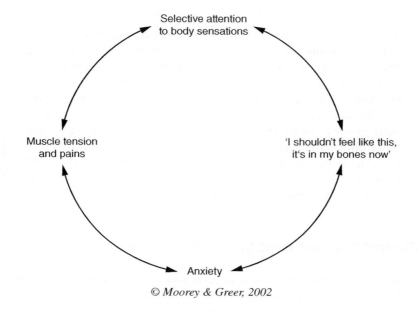

© *Moorey & Greer, 2002*

It does not matter where you start on the circle. Maybe you vaguely notice an ache in the body or perhaps a feeling of background anxiety. Wherever your attention lands, it quickly impacts on other aspects of your system. Anxiety leads to tightness in the chest, a racing heartbeat, sweating, and feelings of agitation and shakiness. Tension results, which is an automatic reaction to unpleasant sensations. This leads to tightness and pain in the body. If this is sustained, a tendency to pay vigilant attention to these sensations will develop - with an inner commentary along the lines of:

'I shouldn't feel like this.'

'Maybe this is a sign of cancer returning.'

This pattern will intensify anxiety, and feed a catastrophic story line, which will lead to more pain and tightening in the body. A vicious cycle will thus build.

Have you ever noticed this sort of pattern?

How might you respond in a way that breaks the links of the vicious circle?

Jeremy had a series of unpleasant scares after his treatment for bowel cancer. When this model was shared with him, he immediately recognized it as something he tended to do. 'But what if the pain in the body is actually the cancer returning?' he said, sounding alarmed. I asked him what might be a wise response. 'I suppose I could decide to leave things for a few days, just to see what happened. Then if the pain continued, I could go to my doctor and get it checked out', he replied. 'How might this be different to what you would normally do?' I asked him. 'I think that remembering the model might change my thoughts about it. I could put some practices in place, instead of becoming obsessed by horrific possibilities', he replied, sounding steadier.

Common Adjustment Styles To Cancer

Some colleagues have proposed a model of adjustment[9] to cancer that is based on the interpretations that each person makes in relation to their emotional and behavioural reactions. They suggest that after the initial period of turmoil, there are five ways[9] that each represent a slightly different view of the threat of cancer.

1 **Resourceful Spirit** – seeing illness as a challenge, developing a positive attitude, taking an active role in recovery, seeking appropriate (but not excessive) information and attempting to live as normal a life as possible.
2 **Avoidance or denial** – minimizing the threat of the illness, holding on to a good prognosis, and letting cancer have as little impact on life as possible.
3 **Fatalism** – passively accepting, believing there is not much that he or she can do (as the patient), so leaves it in the hands of others (the medical professionals) to do what they can.
4 **Helplessness and hopelessness** – feeling overwhelmed by the enormity of the threat of cancer, believing there is nothing they can do to help the situation, basically giving up.
5 **Anxious preoccupation** – constantly searching for reassurance, worrying about possible recurrence, assuming the worst of every physical symptom, and seeing the future as unpredictable.

We are all shaped by our early experiences and formative influences. You may recognize yourself in more than one of the five above. Perhaps at some point you have felt hopeless about the future. There were probably times when you soldiered on as if nothing had happened. A minor physical symptom may leave you feeling intensely anxious, and hunting for information. As time passes, our ways of adjusting and understanding things change, even if we have a predominant style of coping. We are developing ways of building the capacity to respond with awareness in order to support wellbeing and influence events positively as much as possible.

Opening The Fist Of Aversion

Central to Mindfulness-Based Approaches is the principle that it is not necessarily the primary difficulty itself that cause us most trouble, but our reactions to it. If we can gently open to the unwanted, instead of resisting and pushing it away, we can change our relationship to it and radically transform the suffering involved.

There is a simple exercise that demonstrates this. You can do it for yourself:

> *Take a pen and hold it in your hand. Imagine the pen represents a difficulty. Instinctively you will probably tighten around the pen, clenching your fist around it and pushing it away. 'I don't want you'. 'Go away'. Would that we could just drop it, but with a difficulty such as cancer, this is simply not an option.*
>
> *Now, still holding the pen, turn your hand over, and open your fist with your fingers facing upwards. The pen is now lying in your open palm – resistance gone. The pen/the difficulty is still there, it has not gone away, but you can hold it there, without needing to react to it.*

Holding things gently is how we can skilfully respond to difficulty. This is what we are learning to do.

Mapping Emotions In The Body

Recognizing the physical trademarks of emotions is another aid to spotting upcoming emotional weather patterns. Here is a basic and simplified outline of some primary emotions:

Sadness
Often feels *wet*, even if tears are not actually shed. The body might seem to *slump*, with the head and the chest going forwards and curling down. If we try to hide these feelings, we may find ourselves straightening the back, and turning away.

Happiness
In contrast seems to have a *bright, upward* and *outward* energy. If you watch children playing, they jump up and down, often with their arms in the air. When we are happy, we smile or laugh, and seem to radiate happiness. It is hard to miss!

Anger
Can feel *hot*, tight and *hard*. We seem to feel it in the centre of the chest. We may go red in the face, and may clench the fists.

Love
Feels more *warm* and *enfolding*. It also seems to start from the middle of the chest (the heart). There is soft, open quality to love.

Fear
Might be felt *as cold, wobbly,* and *shaky*. When we feel anxious or afraid, we might feel sick or perhaps experience trembling in the limbs.

Calm
Feels more *balanced* with the body seeming to be 'grounded', present and steady.

All these emotions are natural and have their own physiology, which may be experienced differently from person to person. They are natural responses to events and situations, influenced by personal histories, interpretations, and mood. Sadness, fear and anger might be considered 'negative' emotions. In reality, they are simply part of the experience of being alive. The other three – happiness, love and calm – might be seen as 'positive', but are also just feelings that come and go, like emotional 'weather'. We may feel more comfortable with some emotions than others and we are certainly affected by the emotions of others.

Some things to remember

- We all tend to react when stressed and under pressure.
- Becoming familiar with our patterns helps us to learn to interrupt 'automatic' reactivity – and respond differently.
- By pausing and responding mindfully, we change our relationship to what challenges us – and by doing this, the difficulty itself changes.

Short Practices

We have two new short practices that are designed to help you recognize and *respond* when difficulty arises. The first one helps you connect with the felt sense of reactivity in the body. The second practice is a simple breathing space which you can take anywhere with you – to support your capacity to respond when difficulty or unpleasant experience shows up.

The Body Barometer[10]

If you have an old fashioned barometer or have seen one, you will know that you use it by gently tapping on the glass front. Depending on which way the needle moves, it is possible to forecast upcoming weather. We can use our bodies in a similar way to give us sensitive information about upcoming emotional 'weather'.

The body barometer[10]

Here is how you do this:

1 *Determine some part of the body – preferably in the trunk – such as the chest area or the abdomen or somewhere between the two – that for you is especially sensitive to sensations of stress and difficulty. You can put your hand there.*
2 *Once you have found the place, it can become your 'Body Barometer'. Tuning into it regularly, you will notice different sensations at different times. When you are under pressure, feeling anxious, or irritable, you may notice sensations of tension, tightness, shakiness, or discomfort. The intensity of these sensations varies, depending on the level of your difficulty.*

---

3 *As you practice this, you can become aware of quite subtle sensa-*
tions. These may signal that something is just beginning to emerge,
long before you are aware of this in the mind. If you wish, you can
practice Coming to the Breath, or do a Breathing Space to help you
to turn towards and gently 'hold' what is happening. Or you may
choose just to monitor the sensations in your 'barometer', moment by
moment, and be with them as they are.

It only takes a few moments to turn to The Body Barometer to discover what is there. Like so many of the short mindfulness practices, they are easy to practice. The challenge with them all is to remember. How will you remember to check-in to your Body Barometer? Can you set up a reminder specifically for this? If the Pause is now established for you, you might add a Body Barometer onto the end of a Pause? If you can practice this a few times every day for a fortnight, you will establish it as a resource readily available to you.

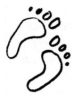

A Breathing Space

This practice will be familiar to you. We have merged a number of practices that you already know. It is easy and accessible, already there 'tucked into your back pocket' and ready to use wherever you are – perhaps when you notice something going on in your Body Barometer.

A breathing space

*Shifting into an upright, relaxed and tall position … … sitting or standing … … and **Pausing** … … just interrupting the flow of your attention and deliberately asking yourself 'What is going on for me right now?' … … … or 'How am I feeling right now?' … … noticing … … then when you are ready, becoming aware of the contact of our **Feet on the Floor** … … and the detailed sensations in the soles of your feet … … lingering there until your attention is fully engaged in your feet on the floor … … … … … Now when you're ready, **Coming to the Breath**, breathing itself deep in the body … … … Perhaps coming up close to the beginnings of the next in-breath … … … … the texture of that breath … … … maybe noticing the little pause between the in-breath and the out-breath … … … Breath breathing in, breath breathing out … … … and if the mind wanders away from the breath at any point, just noticing – remembering that it is not a problem for the mind to wander … … and when you have noticed, gently coming back – to the breath in this present moment … …*

1   *Pausing – Noticing*
2   *Feet on the Floor – Arriving in the Body*
3   *Coming to the Breath – The Anchor into this present moment*

How will you remember to practice this? Your thread might act as a reliable reminder, if you are wearing one. The bead will remind you to practice your Breathing Space. You might set up a daily program by hooking a Breathing Space onto an existing activity – such as:

- waiting for the kettle to boil or the computer to boot up
- before you get out of bed in the morning, as you get into bed at night
- after the end of each meal.

You are encouraged to form an intention to practice a Breathing Space at times that you decide, over the next fortnight or so. Two or three times a day is what is recommended, and remembering that if you do not manage this as you intend, to start again with a new intention of when you *will* practice it. The Breathing Space is a valuable and important short practice that we bring into the 'cancer' practices. Investing the time to establish it over the next weeks will repay you many times over.

Additional Practices

Time in nature

This activity links us to Turning Towards the Lovely. Inviting you to find the energy and incentive to get out and spend time in nature – to walk and notice all the ordinary happenings around you. Perhaps choosing themes to focus on – a colour – the movement of the season – sounds – or the way that birds, animals and insects move and interact. Becoming aware of detail – and then of opening to awareness of spaciousness. Being in nature can be good for us, especially when there is a lot going on internally. The movement of the body, the air on the skin, all your senses experiencing your surroundings – notice how you feel after you have done this. It is worth the effort!

Writing or drawing in nature

If you enjoy writing or drawing, you might want to take your notebook outside with you. At different points, you can pause, sit down and form words or images around what you notice – what you see, hear, and sense. There is no need to censor any idea or imagine you are doing this for anyone other than yourself. Just bring whatever comes into your mind, or attracts your attention, onto the page. Let yourself be inspired and nourished by all that is around you.

The Experience Of Cancer

Living With Uncertainty

The sense of being in charge is always a thin veneer waiting to be cracked like ice on a pond.[1]

In this section, we explore the period immediately after the end of major[11] treatment. We look at the particular challenges of this time, and develop some practices to meet them.

The end of treatment

You have been longing for this day to come – your last day of treatment. And here it is! So why does not feel like the celebration you expected?

The end of treatment can often be emotional and challenging. Up to this point, you have had regular contact with your medical team. Everything has been done to remove the cancer, and reduce the chance of it coming back. Now, you are encouraged to go home and pick up on life. But how do you do that?

Picking up the psychological reins

It is well known that the period following treatment can be psychologically challenging. Family and friends assume it is all finished now. You have come through tough treatments, really bravely – yet internally, you may be feeling alone, and most of all afraid.

Internal judgements may abound. 'How come I feel like this?' 'Why am I not being more positive?' 'What is wrong with me?' 'I feel so anxious'.

These reactions are common. Be reassured that there is nothing wrong with you. You are probably feeling much like other people in your situation. It makes a lot of sense that this is a difficult time. The challenges of treatment are considerable and largely physical, once you were in the swing of them. It was almost as if you could put the worry down, and give it to your medical team. They would keep you safe, and hopefully you trusted them to do their job well.

Now that treatment is over, the emotional and psychological impact of all that you've been through is just beginning. And this is tough. Many of us feel unsupported and on our own. After all those visits to the hospital or the clinic, we now have weeks and days without any appointments at all. No longer is our life carved into regular commitments. No longer do we know what each day will bring.

You may not be feeling well. Treatment may be over but side effects are probably still present. You may feel exhausted and worn out. Treatment can seem a bit like running a marathon, requiring stamina, courage, and endurance. Now you are faced with a transition back into 'ordinary' life. It is hard – but there are things you can do to support this time.

Acknowledging what is here

This is a good first step. Rather than expecting everything to be straightforward and smooth, it might be skilful to prepare for a tricky transition from treatment to after treatment. Planning for this for ourselves is a good first start. Preparing friends and family is also important. They may be tired and emotionally wrung out by all that they have seen you go through. However, it is important for them to realize how demanding this transition can be.

Drawing on existing resources

Although this is different from other experiences, you are bound to have had other stressful transitions. Moving home, changing jobs, having a child all involve major change. Reflect back on how you managed. What were the messages that you gave yourself? What was helpful? Is this something that others can help you with – or ways that you can dig deep into your own resources to support you at this time?

Here are some ideas that others had:

I gave myself more time in bed. I knew I was exhausted, so I got up later and went to bed earlier. It is true, I was not sleeping that well – but even reading in bed, or watching a film on my tablet enabled me to rest up. I did this deliberately for as long as I needed to – and even after I was more myself, I still went back to bed sometimes in the middle of the day when I felt tired or lacking in energy.

I made a point of asking friends for support. I had been quite independent during treatment and had relied mostly on family. So now I contacted friends and suggested we went out somewhere, or to meet me for coffee. It helped me get used to those early days when there seemed to be so much time and so little in my calendar.

I have always been active and fit – and I had been looking forward to taking exercise again. It was harder than I expected. So with the support of a training partner, I slowed down, took it gently, was much kinder to myself, and brought my mindfulness practice into the details of the whole experience. Little by little, as I kept going, I could see and feel some progress.

I went back into the garden. It had been sadly neglected, but I knew I could only do a little at a time. It was quite frustrating, yet at one time I didn't even believe I would get this far. It was spring and a lovely time to be starting again. When the bulbs and plants and flowers came through, I think I enjoyed them more than I ever have done.

I wanted to show some appreciation for the kindness and care that my family had given me. I still felt weak, and often anxious and afraid. Yet in some ways this spurred me on. Having had cancer, I didn't know how long I would live for. Why not make the most of every day? So I planned a holiday that we could all enjoy. I spent ages on the Internet researching it all. It gave me much pleasure and the holiday itself was wonderful.

I spent more time with my grandchildren. Having been so ill, it was such a pleasure just to sit and watch them, and play with them. I did not have to expend lots of energy. They knew I was still not well – but every day I spent with them, was a day I could enjoy. I felt so fortunate to have them in my life – to have my life.

Remission

We all hope that we will never need radical treatment again – but in reality, no one knows what the future will bring. Some people finish treatment with a good prognosis. Others are told that cancer may return. Uncertainty accompanies everyone. Day by day, there will be thoughts rumbling in the background relating to a pain, a cough, and any number of other small symptoms. A television program, a friend's diagnosis, something you read in the newspaper or hear on the news – any of them may trigger spikes of anxiety. The fear that cancer may return is never far away, especially in the early days after treatment. This is what we learn to live with.

The way in which a man accepts his fate and all the suffering it entails … … gives him ample opportunity – even under the most difficult circumstances – to add a deeper meaning to his life.[6]

A Mindful Practice For Uncertainty

A Breathing Space

This practice is exactly the same as the second short practice earlier in this chapter. It is a combination of practices that you are already familiar with, drawn from earlier practices that you have learned. This three-part breathing space is designed to help you respond to whatever is arising, wherever you are and whenever you need it. Many find it invaluable, especially in the context of feeling anxious and managing times of uncertainty and transition.

A breathing space

Shifting into an upright, relaxed and tall position … … sitting or stand-ing … … and **Pausing** *… … just interrupting the flow of your attention and deliberately asking yourself 'What is going on for me right now?' … … … or 'How am I feeling right now?' … … noticing … … then when you are ready, becoming aware of the contact of our* **Feet on the Floor** *… … and the detailed sensations in the soles of your feet … … lingering there until your attention is fully engaged in your feet on the floor … … … … … Now when you're ready,* **Coming to the Breath,** *breathing itself deep in the body … … … Perhaps coming up close to the beginnings of the next in-breath … … … … the texture of that breath … … … maybe noticing the little pause between the in-breath and the out-breath … … … Breath breathing in, breath breathing out … … … and if the mind wanders away from the breath at any point, just noticing – remembering that it is not a problem for the mind to wander … … and when you have noticed, gently coming back – to the breath in this present moment … …*

1   *Pausing – Noticing*
2   *Feet on the Floor – Arriving in the Body*
3   *Coming to the Breath – The Anchor into this present moment*

Hannah had advanced cancer. She had a young daughter Annabelle, who felt upset whenever she had to say goodbye. Hannah was having treatment in a cancer centre some distance away from their home. It involved an overnight stay, so these times were hard for them both. Hannah wore a thread to remind her to practice a breathing space whenever she felt anxious. Annabelle asked if she could have one too. After that, whenever they were apart, they both would touch their threads to connect with each other. It was one of a number of things that helped Annabelle manage that difficult time – and Hannah found it immensely reassuring.

Intention For The 'Month' of Turning Towards

Take as long as you need to work through this chapter – doing this in whatever way serves you best. Here are the practices and approaches for you to follow over this next period.

Practices – for each 2 week period

Core Practice	– Sitting Practice [10+ times]
Short Practices	– The Body Barometer [ideally daily]
	– A Breathing Space [2 or 3 × a day]
Exercise	*Reflecting on an unpleasant experience every day*

Cancer Practice – with the thread

Practice for Uncertainty	– A Breathing Space *whenever needed*

In this chapter, we have been developing the key mindfulness-based movement that responds to difficulty. The first two movements of Intention and Coming Back are the building blocks to get you to this point. They will support you well – and Turning Towards is the radical movement that transforms your relationship to suffering.

Intention

Encouraging you to renew your intention to keep going – to keep learning – to keep practicing. Ask anyone who has benefitted a lot from mindfulness and they will tell.

What really matters to you?
How can you bring that into everyday reality?

Checking your reminders are in place. Continuing to do whatever you are finding is helpful – reflecting in your notebook; nourishing your spirit with nature and beauty and friendship; exploring your inner-ness to use this time well to nurture your well-being. Be sure to appreciate your efforts – day by day, step by step, moment by moment is how we thread mindfulness into our lives.

Notes

1 Gross, K. (2015)
2 Quoted in Chödrön, P. (1991)
3 A practice of turning towards the difficult (mild to moderate) has been included on the companion website for this title.
4 Trigonos, North Wales. www.trigonos.org
5 I first heard 'flooding' as a metaphor used in this way by Akincano Marc Weber in a number of his talks. Available at: www.dharmaseed.org
6 Frankl, V.E. (1959/1984)
7 Thanks to Christina Feldman.
8 Teasdale, J., Williams, M., & Segal, Z. (2014) (p. 132)
9 Moorey, S., & Greer, S. (2012)
10 This used to be known as The Physical Barometer (Bartley, 2012).
11 Radical treatment refers to the treatment process after diagnosis or perhaps recurrence – surgery, radiotherapy, chemotherapy and others. There may be ongoing drug treatments, which are taken at home or involve a short visit to the oncology clinic.

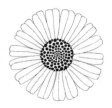

Personal Story

Peter

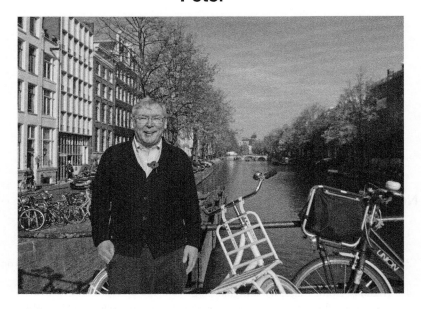

Peter is 67 and married to his childhood sweetheart V, who he met when he was 19. They have a daughter. Peter took early retirement because he felt unwell and was then diagnosed with prostate cancer. He has always been a keen cyclist and fell walker. He loves to read and is interested in Buddhism. He has a very dry sense of humour!

Mindfulness: A Kindly Approach to Being with Cancer, First Edition. Trish Bartley.
© 2017 John Wiley & Sons, Ltd. Published 2017 by John Wiley & Sons, Ltd.
Companion Website: www.wiley.com/go/bartley/mindfulness

Diagnosis

I was diagnosed with prostate cancer on St Valentine's Day, two years ago. The urologist told me rather bluntly. His first language wasn't English, so it came as a brutal shock. V was there, of course. She had already guessed. I'd had tests and biopsies and the PSA test had come back sky-high. My father had died from cancer, which we later suspected had originated in the prostate. On our return from a family funeral of a relative who had died from prostate cancer, there were two urgent messages on the answer machine saying you must get in touch with your doctor immediately.

I was devastated. It felt like being hit in the gut with a 5 lb hammer. He was a good guy, the urologist, and a good clinician, but his language wasn't subtle. I said, 'Is it cancer'? And he said, 'yes it is' – just like that. Apparently he said that I would be treated with injections and radiotherapy – but I don't remember that. I went completely blank. I think I was in shock for quite some days. This led to an ongoing depression. I was staying awake at night, constantly playing a tape in my head. It was the end of the game. I was going to die of this cancer.

What it also did was bounce me off my meditation. I had started meditating intermittently in the 70s. They called it transcendental meditation. It cost me a lot of money to get a mantra, and I promptly forgot it! So I just concentrated on the breath. But once I was diagnosed, I completely forgot about my practice.

A few weeks later, I read an article in the newspaper about mindfulness. Then I went onto YouTube and saw Jon Kabat-Zinn. I did a bit of research and discovered there were MBSR courses you could go to. I booked up and went on a five-day intensive course soon after, run by Bangor University.

Treatment

I had eight weeks of radiotherapy treatment. This started about six months after diagnosis. The main reaction was an all-consuming fatigue – both physical and mental. This lasted for quite a while, but that could be related to the Parkinson's that I've got.

The staff at the radiotherapy centre were absolutely magnificent. We met the same people every day. We gave them a huge cake at the end, which they quite appreciated. Of course, I had to show my bits to the world when I had the radiotherapy. It was just a job that had to be done. But I felt as if I was getting world-class treatment. I'd been told that it was state-of-the-art. I made the best of it really.

I've also had injections every three months. I had the first, the day I was diagnosed and I have the last one next February. There is a hormone in the injections, which reduces my testosterone levels. As a result of these, my libido vanished. This happened straight away. I was warned – but speaking as a vigorous male, it is devastating. It is all bound up with your self-image and your masculinity. I think it was a major cause of the depression – the lack of maleness and potency.

But over time you adapt and seem to care less about it – and you have to shave less often – so it's not all bad news! As a couple, we just make the best of it. It is important to keep talking. A male thing to do is to go into your cave and roll a boulder over the door. It's important to keep expressing how it feels – and how you feel about one another. We like a cuddle now and again. Just because I've lost my libido, it doesn't mean there is no physical contact between us.

Mindfulness

By the time I had radiotherapy, my mindfulness practice was back on track. I was doing 20 minutes, sitting on a stool – sometimes a guided meditation, and sometimes just concentrating on the breath.

I found my practice helped me in accepting the diagnosis. It helped me manage the rumination, and the low mood and anxiety. It helps to live in the moment and experience life as enhancing each moment – that's a quote you will have heard a few times before! That sounds rather pretentious, but it just seems ordinary for me to meditate. If I don't do it, I miss it – and I am super lucky to have V, who is a meditator and C, my daughter, who is as well. So if my practice falls off, I get gentle reminders from my family and my friend P as well.

I practice in the morning, either before or after breakfast. During the day, I use my thread[12] for automatic negative thoughts. For example, when we had a break away recently, there was bad fog on the day we were due to fly home. V said that we'd land ok, but I thought we would probably have to be diverted miles away. As soon as I noticed that I'd moved into my pattern of negative thinking, I just held on to my bead. It offers me a moment of respite and recollection. I recognize the negative thought, and I just hold the bead for a few seconds. It works! First, I acknowledge that it is just an automatic negative thought and then it just dissolves away.

I would advise anyone in a similar position – just do it (*practice mindfulness*). Just sit and don't look for results or improvements. Don't self-monitor and it will happen. You will have a calmer, gentler, and more loving outlook on life.

Parkinson's disease

I was diagnosed with Parkinson's just after finishing my radiotherapy. I'd had a slight tremor for some time, which is not a handy thing to have if you are a dentist! You have to laugh – you might as well. I decided to retire – but I was not actually diagnosed until two years later. I got the cancer diagnosis and the Parkinson's diagnosis in the same year. Luckily I didn't get anything the following year!

I think I'm having more difficulty with the Parkinson's now than the prostate. With the prostate you accommodate to it. Parkinson's is a degenerative disease. It is easy to fall into rumination about the long-term effects. That is another good reason to keep meditating. If I didn't have Parkinson's, life would be a lot better.

I don't want to sound self-pitying, but the major thing about mindfulness is acceptance. It is the same with any disease. Once you can accept that these are the cards you've been dealt, it's a lot easier to get on with life, and enjoy life. But if you rail against it, it makes life difficult. Sometimes I fall into it, the self-pity – and then I'll have a moment of recollection. I use mindfulness as a form of therapy at times, if I start to feel sorry for myself – which is a futile emotion to have. When that happens, I will go to my stool and sit – or just sit upright in a chair for five minutes or so.

The future

My cancer prognosis is pretty good but I am coming to the end of my treatment and I think at some time in the future the cancer will start to grow again. When that happens I will have further treatment, but I think it will be palliative.

They monitor the dormancy of the cancer through a PSA test. They are always very positive when they talk to me about it, but I don't explore it with them. They tell me that the PSA levels are low, then they try and leave it and I don't push them.

It interests me that the long-term future with cancer doesn't have much impact on me now. I think I've come to terms with it. It can be pretty devastating when you get the diagnosis. Then in time and with mindfulness practice, I think you just learn to cope. I wouldn't say it's gone completely. It's always at the back of my mind, but it gives life more of a frisson, in a way.

I think that I appreciate life more now because of the cancer. I've never got to the point of welcoming it – I stop short of that. I said this to a mate of mine a few months ago, and he looked at me as if I was barmy – the idea that you could welcome cancer. On a day-to-day basis, Parkinson's definitely affects me more, because of the pain and the lack of mobility. It also affects my speed of thinking, which is the most distressing aspect of all.

As long as I can keep a positive view, and see it as a challenge, I hope I'll be able to keep my nerve, if or when the PSA levels start going up again. I don't think that's any different from anyone else. It's important to me to face that challenge in the light of having a daughter and wife. I want to do the best I can, with their help and strength.

What matters most to me is to be a good role model for my daughter – to let her learn that we are all going to face it at one time or another, and that her old man can face it with dignity and pride. That will be true right up to the end – unless I lose my nerve, and go to pieces – and then I'll pick myself up again.

Note

12 www.thoughtonathread.co.uk – the same as the threads used in this book

Chapter 4
Kindness

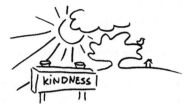

Mindfulness is not a magic wand or an end in itself, but the platform where understanding begins – where healing of that which is broken is possible … Transformation begins with having empathy for our own struggles – our heart trembling in the face of difficulty rather than moving into judgment – which we do so fast.

Christina Feldman[1]

Kindness is the last of our four movements – yet it has been there all along. It is right at the heart of Intention. It is integral to the way of Coming Back. Without gentleness in Turning Towards, we risk becoming tight or driven. Kindness is the medicine that transforms our struggles.

In this chapter, we explore how to cultivate the seeds of kindness and uncover the part that kindness has been playing all along. We learn some new short practices, review those that you have been practicing and give attention to thoughts and how best to manage them. In the final section, we consider how to live with cancer in the longer term, and how to manage an episode of recurrence. There are some dedicated thread exercises that many people value.

Mindfulness is no longer new, even for those of you who were mindfulness 'novices' at the beginning of this book. You have been developing your practice. As we include this last movement of kindness, it is important to remind ourselves of the other three and how they build on each other.

Intention supports us to:

- remember what really matters to us, and
- translate this into everyday actions.

Mindfulness: A Kindly Approach to Being with Cancer, First Edition. Trish Bartley.
© 2017 John Wiley & Sons, Ltd. Published 2017 by John Wiley & Sons, Ltd.
Companion Website: www.wiley.com/go/bartley/mindfulness

Coming back helps us to:

- bring attention to gently explore present moment experience
- notice when the mind wanders
- choose wisely rather than react automatically.

Turning towards enables us to:

- allow what is present to gently be as it is
- remember our tendencies of fight or flight
- choose to gently turn towards the felt sense in the body; OR wisely find another place to stand
- connect with what is lovely - another way of being with difficulty.

Qualities of mindfulness

Many people assume that mindfulness is solely about training attention. Some people believe that it is a way of clearing the mind. These views limit an understanding of the depth, scope, and potential that mindfulness offers us for being skilfully engaged in our lives.

With diligent practice, mindfulness enables us to learn to slow down. Instead of rushing on, there is now possibility of pausing and noticing what is happening. We are learning to be curious – to explore what is here. Mindfulness is a bit like a light beam illuminating either the detail of what we choose to attend to, or widening into more spacious awareness. From time to time, we notice that the mind wanders off into thoughts, fantasies and ruminations. With practice we remember to come back to the breath and the body, in the immediacy of present moment experience.

This brief overview of mindfulness may be in line with your experience, but it seems a little dry. There is not much warmth in there. Any worthwhile description of mindfulness will include its 'relational' qualities, such as kindness and compassion. We know this on an intellectual level, but may find it challenging to bring it into life. When we have experienced the effect of kindness in practice for ourselves, then we can cultivate these qualities to grow within us.

Awareness … … of inner mental states is not enough; people also need kindness to recruit resources in themselves that are imaginative, nurturing and empowering.[2]

Connecting In Kindness

We generally associate kindness with how we behave towards others. It might show itself through the love we offer a friend. Love usually asks to be recip- rocated. We can feel hurt when our feelings are not shared.

Kindness is a quality within mindfulness that has the manner of profound friendliness. Unlike some forms of love, it needs nothing back.

It is important to understand that we are making no distinction here between responding kindly to our own experience and being kind to someone else. In fact, you might practice kindness by deliberately asking yourself at times, 'Would I treat others like this?' This might make you pause for thought for there is an ethical component here. Can it ever be right to habitually treat some- one unkindly? We tend to be blind to the dishonesty of giving kindness to others yet ignoring and devaluing being gentle towards ourselves.

Being self-compassionate or kind in response to our own distress has little part in Western mainstream culture. Many of us instinctively baulk at it – believing it to sound selfish, 'flaky', self-indulgent or self-absorbed. However, we are not referring to some shallow tokenistic approach here – nor is it more natural to women than men.

Kindness is a quality that naturally includes, connects and befriends – whether practiced with one's own experience, or offered to another. It is integral to the cultivation of mindfulness practice and mindful living.

Arthur was puzzled by the invitation to soften into sensations in the body, in order bring kindness into his practice. A quiet and gentle man, he worked as a vet before being diagnosed with cancer. In response to his bewilderment, we tried a number of ways to approach this feeling of kindness, but Arthur remained mystified.

At the end of the session, we headed outside. As I let my dog out of the car, Arthur immediately bent down and greeted him with, 'Hello lovely!' His movement towards the dog, his interest in him, the tone of his voice, his touch and even his eye contact oozed with kindness. There it was! This was the feeling he could 'borrow' when connecting to kindness in his practice.

Compassion is sister to kindness. It is a response to pain, distress, or difficulty – a hurt child; a family member going through tough times; or someone in the chemo ward looking upset. It might involve a generous act; a thoughtful gesture; or simply holding the other in heart and mind. Compassion is kindness in the face of suffering that has no thought of wanting something back. We probably know these feelings for others, but rarely extend them to our own pain and suffering.

The good news is that the potential for kindness and compassion is something we all have within us – both when extended to others and in relation to ourselves. Some would say that it is what makes us essentially human. It is the glue that gathers the qualities of mindfulness together. It is the ground in which our practice thrives.

We each need to connect with a capacity to befriend our experience – to find our own doorway into the kindness of the heart – for it is this that frees us.

Obstacles and invitations to kindness

The curious paradox is that when I accept myself just as I am, then I can change.[3]

When we react with impatience to old habits – tightening around them, disliking and judging them – reacting like any hurt creature – we close up and defend. When we manage to turn towards these same patterns in openness and understanding, there is a softening response that resonates within the body. These tiny gestures can have profound impact.

There are many moments in the day when we move into reactivity, with harshness and contraction in the mind. Mindfulness is rightly termed a practice. It needs remembering over and over, as if wearing a groove in the body mind, so that our habits of unkindness are replaced, little by little, with moments of awareness that open naturally into kindly habits.

A group of young psychologists on a mindfulness course were finding things hard. They wanted to discover the 'right' way to 'do' mindfulness. I wrote to them after one of our sessions. Here is an excerpt from my email:

You are learning to BE with yourself – and most of us find this very difficult at first … You have been told that mindfulness isn't another fix, yet somehow we all hope that it is.

You can't 'do' mindfulness in the ways that have worked for you before. The hard work needed now is to practice with gentleness. Can you see what happens if you experiment with adding a few drops of patience to the next body scan? Or little traces of kindness as you practice a breathing space? Using effortless effort, knowing there is no right way. Caring a lot, but without any goal. Practicing as if your life depends on it, yet just doing it every day!

It is not surprising that having worked so hard to pass their exams and get on in the world, they would bring the same goal oriented approach to learning mindfulness. The problem is that this way of doing things can result in anxiety, resentment and disconnection. We are all at the mercy of feeling good when things go well, and miserable when they do not.

Patterns of mind

Indeed, we seem to be hard wired to want things certain ways. For instance, many of us experience considerable pain and discomfort when having bloods taken. After a few weeks or months, our veins seem to refuse to cooperate, and we dread the next time.

We probably favour one staff member over another. A previously difficult experience may leave us not wanting a certain nurse. We wait in the phlebotomy queue hoping not to get the one we mistrust – so that when we land up in her chair, we anticipate the worst. She tells us to relax, and this simply adds irritation to the mix. It is easy to put the blame on the hapless nurse who hurts us. However, our reactivity in resisting and tightening around the experience will have added to our suffering.

We tend to see life written in permanent ink: 'It is always like that', 'I am always like this' and we judge ourselves in ways a good friend never would. We have such distorted self-images. We spot this in others, but may be blind to our own.

As our awareness grows, we learn that some of our habitual automatic reactions can make things worse. Yet reacting in these ways is entirely human and normal. It is what we tend to do.

Sitting with difficulty

Let us explore this further through a story located in another familiar context. It illustrates that being present with suffering, without trying to change it or make it better, can be a helpful response.

> Jasmine had to have an unpleasant treatment once a month. She dreaded it. One of her friends always came with her. In March, Carole took her to hospital and brought puzzles, stories to read out loud, snacks and all sorts of things to distract them and pass the time. In April, it was Simon's turn. He sat quietly beside the bed. Whenever Jasmine turned to him, Simon was there. She sensed his calm kindness, and found his presence immensely comforting and steadying.

Of course, sitting quietly is not always the most appropriate support. Different situations call for different responses. However, this story illustrates that being fully present, in a way that is receptive and kindly, can be profoundly caring. So often, we try to avoid what is unpleasant by filling the space with busyness. There are better alternatives, we are learning.

Cultivating The Seeds Of Kindness

When I lived in South Africa, I drove into town once a week to post my letters and shop. There was always a long queue in the post office. Early on, I noticed a woman behind the counter, who had a miserable looking face. Over the weeks, I made a bet with myself: Could I get her to smile at me? I failed every week.

It dawned on me one day in the queue – What if this woman looked as she did because was deeply unhappy? My attitude changed immediately. Internally I started to wish her well. Eventually, she served me and smiled … … Her whole face lit up and mine probably did too in response. I was so surprised and happy – and for the rest of that day, I kept remembering that smile. What a gift it was!

From this unremarkable story, we can draw some threads. Kindness at best seems to be:

- unconditional – without goal
- spontaneous – offered in the moment
- heartful – not rational or contrived
- involving connection – not 'self' motivated
- befriending – without thought of getting anything back.

We all have seeds of kindness within us. No big push is required for them to emerge. All that is needed is for the layers of avoiding and holding on to gently dissolve. It is like the sun, always there behind the clouds. When the clouds clear, the sun shines through, giving warmth and light. So it is with kindness. Can we practice by forming an intention to open to the warmth of kindness, whenever we feel contracted in the body?

Mindfulness practice helps us to view those unwanted parts of ourselves with a softer gaze. In time, we can bring both our strengths and our difficulties into the even warmth of the kind old sun. The capacity to befriend experience starts with tiny movements, little openings and gestures – softening into a pain here; gently bringing the mind back there. Gradually we wake up to how different life can be when we relate to our experience with kindness and compassion, rather than judging and tightening around what is difficult.

Jeremy was having his second chemotherapy, when an allergic reaction caused him to feel extremely ill. Nurses rushed to his side and quickly pushed him across the room to the oxygen. In the middle of this commotion, Jeremy opened his eyes and saw the frightened faces of the others in the treatment room. He registered their alarm and after it was all over, felt sorry that he had given them such a shock.

Some days later, he reflected that none of it was his fault. With this insight came deep compassion for himself. He told me that he felt his heart open. 'It was such a terrifying thing to happen', he said, 'but I realize now that what I saw in those faces was not just shock for themselves, but also concern for me. I feel quite tender towards all of us who have to go through these treatments.

This change of heart made a big difference to Jeremy's experience of subsequent treatments. He felt much more connected with the others having treatment with him. 'They are just like me', he felt when he looked at them.

There is nothing hackneyed about self-compassion or kindness. There are no soft violins, clichéd phrases, or pink and white ribbons – just an awareness that is allowing, forgiving and opening. Feelings of poignancy and tenderness often release. This is not sadness as such, but the heart opening through layers of contraction and defendedness.

Reaching out

When we recognize and connect with the pain of others, we naturally want to reach out. It somehow resonates in us in a way that can touch us deeply.

In all our individual states, we are always communal. There is always a point where one hand reaches out to another.[4]

Can we reach out to ourselves in the same way? We yearn for connectedness. Can you connect with those parts of yourself that you dislike? Can you open in kindness for all the challenges you have faced through being ill?

I remember teaching someone who proudly told me that she had not cried once since being diagnosed. After a day of mindfulness practice, she went home and cried for several hours. Her family was concerned, but she regretted none of it, she said, 'It is like a heavy weight has lifted off my shoulders.'

Meeting ourselves with compassion

We have subtly folded kindness and compassion into all the practices we have followed thus far. We have done this carefully so as not to overwork things, or use kindness as a Band-Aid, which covers over the tender places, but does not really attend to them.

Living with cancer, becoming vulnerable and needing help brings these tender places into light. We have to rely on others in new ways. It can be as challenging to be vulnerable and accept help, as it is to relate kindly to your own illness, pain and distress. However, there are also other aspects to being vulnerable that can serve as opportunities for compassionate practice.

When Derek was diagnosed with a rare cancer, he had to go for specialized surgery, at the other end of the country. During his lengthy recovery in hospital, he received many cards from friends back home. 'I spent time reflecting on love and kindness in my hospital bed and realized just how powerful it is. I felt strongly connected to a sense of goodness in the world', he said. Later, he developed his own way of using kindness phrases with the breath. This became the basis of his practice. 'I now have the chance to be thoughtful in a positive way', he told me, 'both towards myself and towards others.'

Could you develop your own kindness phrases? You may remember them from the additional waiting and treatment practices. You might add a phrase or two to the beginning and end of your sitting practice – and repeat them internally to yourself during the day. Many people find this extraordinarily helpful.

Here are some examples that you can adapt and change:

May I be safe and protected.
May I live with love and kindness.
May I be as well as it is possible for me to be.
May I be content.
May I be peaceful and have ease of heart and mind.

You can personalize them – allowing them to relate more closely to your personal circumstances, by adding 'in the midst of ... ...'.

Here are some ideas:

May I be safe and protected, in the midst of fear and uncertainty.
May I live with kindness, in the midst of busyness.
May I be as well as it is possible for me to be, in the midst of cancer and illness.
May I be content and appreciative, in the midst of difficulty and challenge.
May I be peaceful and have ease of heart and mind, in the midst of conflict.

Developing ways of bringing kindness into your day might start before your feet touch the ground first thing in the morning, with a gentle noticing of how you are. You might finish the day with resting your head on the pillows, feeling the bed linen around you, and repeating to yourself, 'May I rest well'. In the 'empty' waiting moments – while the kettle is coming to the boil, or the computer is booting up – there are many opportunities to pause and come back to the body, and bring kindly awareness to however things are.

Sometimes it can feel strange to connect kindly with different parts of the body, especially where we have had treatment:

At first, Enid was nervous of bringing attention to where she had had surgery. To start with, she just ignored it. Then in one practice, she tentatively had a go – and was *surprised* to find no special sensation there. Over time, she could linger there and breathe into it, sending kindly thoughts to the whole area. 'It feels good somehow', she said.

Eventually, we seek to cultivate kindness for all aspects of our pain, whether physical or emotional. For example, if you have pain in your knee, you would first practice bringing gentle awareness to the pain itself – then you would extend kindness into the whole of the knee – and finally to the part of you that does not want the pain.

Finally, here is a story of a young woman who connected to a practice that meant the world to her.

Barbara was in her mid-30s, with a young family, when diagnosed with advanced cancer. It was a tragedy for them. Barbara called on many sources of support including mindfulness to help her manage. She was especially fond of mountain practice. It reminded her of the day her husband proposed to her, halfway up a mountain. She would practice using the image of the mountain, until she felt more grounded and steady. Then she would imagine that she was sitting on the top of a mountain with a vast spacious view all around. From there, she offered out love to everyone below, imagining it radiating out to her partner and children, and coming back to her – to her parents and siblings, to her friends, and out into the world – radiating out and back, out and back.

We begin to find that, to the degree that there is bravery in ourselves – the willingness to look, to point directly at our own hearts – and the degree that there is kindness towards ourselves, there is confidence that we can actually forget ourselves and open to the world"[5].

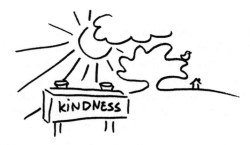

Practices And Understandings

In this section we look at some new practices; review the previous chapter's practices; explore the Unpleasant Experience Exercise and further our understanding of thoughts and how to relate to them.

Review thus far

Moving on now to ask:
Am I remembering to integrate practice with everyday life?
When I develop an approach that is helpful, am I bringing it through into the learning of the next section?
How am I adapting practices to make them my own?

Many of you reading this book might assume that the way I describe things is the only way – or the best way to do them. This is not necessarily so. I would encourage you to be creative, especially once you have the building blocks in place. You know what works best for you – so adapt, experiment and discover ways that support you best.

New Practices

Core Practices   – Walking with Kindness, or
                             – Customizing your core practice with kindness
                                included
Short Practices   – Coming to the Breath with kindness
                             – Three Step Breathing Space

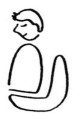

Core Practice

It is helpful to decide in advance how long you will walk for – perhaps choosing to walk for 15 minutes or so. You may notice that if you leave the time open, it is all too easy to find yourself stopping, whenever you get bored or distracted. Walking through those moments and reconnecting with your intention to practice, helps you sustain your intentional awareness, and resist the reactive pull to avoid some things and attach to others.

Walking with kindness

1 Start by **Standing in Mountain** – *outside if possible. Feeling your feet on the ground. Setting up the body … Weight going down, rooted to the earth beneath … … Height going up, connecting with the sky above … … Standing like a mountain, tall and dignified … Now pausing and checking in, 'What is going on for me right now?'*

2 *Framing an **intention** to practice walking with kindness – and **bring someone to mind**. Choosing a person with whom you have no special history, who you associate with kindliness – perhaps a teacher, a mentor, a neighbour, or even a pet.*

3 *Choosing a track or pathway to walk along – 10 or so steps either way – and imagining that your kindly person is standing beside you – perhaps with a hand tucked under your arm.*

When you are ready, setting off to walk mindfully. Once your mindful walking is established, bring attention to your 'imaginary companion', and feeling their kindness towards you … … … offering him/her some kindly phrases as you walk together. 'May you be peaceful'. 'May you be happy'. 'May you have ease of heart and mind'. Seeing how this feels … … … continuing to walk mindfully, slowly up and down your track, pausing at the ends, and repeating the phrases now and again. Let yourself connect with a sense of kindness from your imaginary companion, and offering kindness and appreciation to them in turn.

I looked out over the retreat room, and outside into grounds below – and could see people silently engrossed in walking practice, many with right arms bent, as if someone's hand was tucked into theirs. It was moving to see.

Later, in the feedback, a number of people spoke. 'I went for a walk with Dad. He died 3 months ago', a middle-aged man told us. Several people had extended their practice beyond the original guidance. Someone described 'walking' with a friend she had fallen out with. Many said they found the practice comforting and peaceful.

As with the other core practices, you are encouraged to follow this at least 10 times over the next few weeks – or 20 times over the month. This level of practice commitment will help you to embed the practice into your experience, and will enable you to adapt it to follow in your own way. When that happens, we seem to absorb the practice differently and own it for ourselves.

You might want to follow the guided practice a few times, to help you connect to the quality of kindness – but as you get more familiar with it, you can follow the practice without guidance. We are cultivating a quality of befriending. It needs time and practice, because for most of us this is very new.

Remember that there is no result to aim for. You may not feel much kindness as you practice. You may even feel quite irritated or not feel anything much at all. As best you can, just keep following the guidance on the practice and being curious about your experience and open to what you discover, if anything.

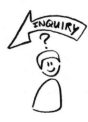

Reflective inquiry

What was happening for you as you practiced Walking with Kindness? What did you notice, in general, and more specifically?

How was it to experience walking in this way?

Customizing your Core Practice

We now take time to review all the core practices. We started with the Body Scan, and then learnt Mindful Walking, and finally we followed Sitting Practice. What have you discovered?

Does one practice suit some moods or situations more than others?
Have you a firm favourite?
Are there any that you dislike, or have not practiced much?
Is it possible to draw any conclusions from this review?
What are you learning about yourself?

Michelle loves the Body Scan. It is what she turns to whenever she feels anxious. When that tight knot arrives in her upper abdomen, she reaches for the recording on her phone. She finds it surprisingly steadying to lie still and move her attention into the detail of physical sensations, even if her mind keeps wandering. 'Just doing it seems to have benefit', she says.

Peter likes to walk, focusing on the soles of his feet and the contact with the ground. He enjoys feeling his footfall – and all the detail of toes, balls of the feet and heels coming into contact with the ground at different times. It gives him a lot to concentrate on. Even if he is feeling tired and flat, he finds that after walking for ten minutes or so, he often feels clearer and more energized.

Annie strongly disliked the sitting practice. It was too static, she said. However, months down the line, she decided to give it another go – and found to her surprise, that she came to love the different sections and how they built one on another. She felt nourished after sitting for a while, even if her mind was scattered at the start. 'I cannot imagine a day without it now', she said.

Over the next month, you are encouraged to see what you are drawn to practice on different days. You might want to mix and match – perhaps starting with a period of Walking with Kindness, and then moving to parts of the Sitting Practice or to the Body Scan. What is important now is to find ways of folding kindness into your practice.

Can you cultivate your intention to be more compassionate to your body and mind, especially in relation to any places of pain, tenderness, anxiety or tightness?
Can you see if it is possible to bring kindliness to the breath, as it breathes? How does this feel?

Practice in these ways as an experiment, with curiosity – without expecting any result.

I came down from the mountain and sat with a mug of tea, my face turned up to the sun. A gentle wind was moving the firs high above me. I closed my eyes to open into the panorama of sound. After a while thoughts lazily appeared – 'shall I plant more trees', 'what to cook for lunch' – and coming back without much effort to the song of the fir trees, mimicking a languid sea.

Short Practices

Coming to the Breath with Kindness

You are already familiar with the beginning of this practice, Coming to the Breath – so inviting you to follow it in a way that suits you, and then adding kindness in on the breath. Once you are familiar with it, and can guide yourself, you can choose how long you want to practice for – from several breaths to a few minutes (or as long as choose).

Coming to the Breath with kindness

Bringing awareness to your feet on the floor ... the feel of your body in contact with the chair ... Weight going down ... Connecting with a sense of your spine rising up ... tall ... dignified ... Height going up.

Then realizing that you are breathing ... Letting the breath breathe itself ... Simply feeling the sensations of the breath deep in the body. If at any point, you notice that your mind has wandered away from the breath ... remembering that this is not a problem – and gently coming back to the anchor of the breath ... breathing in and breathing out.

Now, inviting kindness to flow in on the breath ... ... letting it circulate throughout the whole of your body ... filling every corner and crevice ....Flowing over any tender place ... ... kindness emanating from the heart, flowing into the whole of the body mind like a soft breeze.

Coming to the Breath with Kindness is not complicated. The step of bringing kindness in on the breath is really just an intentional movement of opening gently to your experience in the body and the mind. It is a favourite mindfulness practice of many mindfulness practitioners who have/have had cancer.

- There is no need to feel anything special.
- Not to worry if you have no awareness of kindness.
- It is enough to bring an intention to include kindness.

As with the other short practices, you might choose to practice it once or twice daily, for two weeks or more. Persevering for this long, as best you can, will enable you to ensure it is part of your practice repertoire. We are only able to access practices, if they are already embedded in the body mind. Two weeks of daily practice will probably enable you practice Coming to the Breath with Kindness whenever you need it – providing it remains a fairly regular part of your practice. We easily forget things – but they return fairly readily, if they were once well known to us.

I noticed I had moved into some nasty judging of myself, so I came to the breath with kindness.

Alan (51)

A three step responding space (3SRS)[6]

In the last chapter, we learnt to practice a simple breathing space. If you got on well with it, then do continue. If you would like to develop it a bit further, here is an opportunity. The 3SRS is very accessible. Many people rely on this practice as their number one tool in managing everyday difficulty.

A three step responding space (3SRS)[7]

Before starting the three steps, shift your position in some way. You may choose to do this breathing space by standing in mountain if you want – or sitting on a chair with your feet well planted, knowing the contact with the floor – and choosing to have your eyes open or closed.

Step 1 Noticing
*In the first step, **practicing the Pause** – asking 'What is going on for me right now?' Then extending it, by noticing and acknowledging thoughts … … what feelings are current? … … and then coming into the body, and finding the **Body Barometer**, and noticing … … What physical sensations are here?*

We are just noticing here – not exploring the detail of things, but finding and acknowledging whatever is here.

Step 2 Gathering
*In the second step, **Coming to the Breath** … gathering the attention to the breath breathing deep in the body, rising and falling … You can place a hand on the belly, if you like, to connect with the movement of the breath under your hand … … … If the mind wanders, remembering it is not a problem … and gently coming back to the breath deep in the body, and to the anchor of the present moment, breath by breath.*

Step 3 Expanding
*In the third step, **expanding awareness** around the breath to include a sense of the body as a whole, and the breath breathing within the whole of the body … … breathing body … … Then, opening up a space of awareness beyond the body and the breath, to include whatever is here – and **breathing with it all with kindness**. Saying to yourself gently, if you want to, 'It is ok. Whatever it is, let me feel it'… … and breathing the breath with it all.*

The 3SRS is a skilful way to respond to difficulty. Perhaps a tricky thought arrives, or some emotional reactivity, or maybe a pain in the body that is accompanied by alarming thoughts – then a 3SRS is a way of noticing, coming back and gently holding whatever is there. Remember that when we relate kindly to what is difficult, the experience itself changes.

The 3SRS contains three practices and therefore may take a bit longer to learn and integrate. The first two steps are already familiar – The Pause and Coming to the Breath. The third step is a movement that you practice in the Body Scan and also in the Sitting Practice. This involves moving from one-pointed attentiveness (to the details of the breath), to a wider, more spacious awareness – first into the whole body, and then wider still into whatever is there.

This 'open focus' is a skilful way of holding experience lightly but surely, as it comes and goes, always changing. If this was a landscape you are looking at, you would be seeing land and sky, colours and movements and so on – not focusing on any particular part, but able to scan and appreciate the whole view. In 'panoramic' or spacious awareness, it is similar. We hold the aspects of experience such as emotions, physical sensations, strands of thoughts and storylines as they come and go – not focusing on any one of them, but letting them come and go in the wider container of awareness.

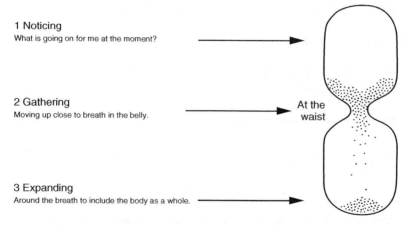

1 Noticing
What is going on for me at the moment?

2 Gathering
Moving up close to breath in the belly.

At the waist

3 Expanding
Around the breath to include the body as a whole.

It helps to remember that this practice has the 'signature' shape of an hourglass. It starts wide at the first step, with pausing and noticing whatever is there – then narrows to the waist (and the detail of the breath) on the second step – and then widens again to hold whatever is there, on the third.

The 3SRS can be followed initially from the guided practice – and once familiar, you can practice it on your own. Practice this daily for a few weeks – so that you have it securely in place available as a resource tool whenever you need it.

Additional Practice

Everyday kindness

Earlier in this chapter, you heard about Derek who uses kindness phrases during the day, internally repeating them to himself.

Similar to the phrases we have used before, this offers you the possibility of using the phrases on their own – for yourself, your loved ones, people you may be having difficulties with, and even those you don't know, who you've seen on the news, or in the hospital. It is always best to practice this for yourself first, before extending them to others. As we have discussed, it is all too easy to focus on others and ignore our own needs for kindness and appreciation.

Choose one of the phrases and repeat it now and again to yourself, as you go about your day. On another day, you may choose a different one. Developing this according to your mood, the events around you, and what is on your mind.

Here are some examples:

May I find kindness in the midst of judgement
May I feel steady in the midst of uncertainty
May I find things to appreciate in the midst of dark times
May I find compassion in the midst of pain and distress

When extending these to others, you simply change the pronoun:

*May **you** find steadiness in the midst of fear – or May **we all** find steadiness in the midst of fear etc.*

Or saying someone's name to yourself :

Tom, may you be safe in this difficult time – Jane, may you find peace in the midst of what you are dealing with.

William's feet were sore after several courses of chemotherapy. He told me that he had never paid much attention to them. This changed and he started looking after them, putting on soothing cream each day. He enjoyed the difference this made. It felt nurturing. When Christmas came, his partner bought him a reflexology session. He and his teenage son, Scott, went together. They loved it. It was a great success – but Scott made his father promise that he would never tell anyone what they had been doing!

Grounded In The Earth

I came feeling that I carried the world on my shoulders,
I leave knowing that it is the earth that carries me.

I came thinking that awareness of the mind was important,
I leave knowing that awareness of the body is indispensable.

I came as a follower of my thoughts,
I leave in the service of my heart.

Pete

Home Practice Review

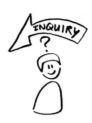

Sitting Practice Review

Reflective inquiry

What are you noticing when you follow the Sitting Practice? What general observations can you make? Inviting you to reflect on your experience, using similar questions to before.

What have you noticed about your experience of the Sitting Practice over this time?
How has that been for you?
What do you make of that, if anything?

If you prefer – you can reflect internally or in your notebook:

What is new in my learning since starting this practice?
What am I discovering about myself, if anything?

The Breath

As we progress through this approach, and having spent time on the sitting practice, you will have noticed that the breath and the body take on an increasingly significant role. We learn to stay close to the breath and this offers us a lot. The breath provides a reliable place to come back to, when the mind wanders off into thoughts; it generates detailed sensations that we can bring friendly curiosity to; and it offers rhythmical dynamic movement within the body that we can rest attention onto. These ways of attending to the breath help to support emotional balance and offer the potential for kindly awareness, within present moment experience.

Cultivating detailed awareness of the breath

It is valuable for each of us to find ways of getting engaged and interested in the sensations of breathing. To facilitate this, we can choose to focus on a particular part of the breath – such as the very beginnings of the next in breath – experiencing this with fresh inquiring attention, as if for the first time.

There are many other parts of the breath that we can pay special attention to at different times:

- the beginning of the in breath
- the flow of the in breath
- the end of the in breath
- the pause at the top
- the beginning of the out breath
- the releasing flow of the out breath
- the end of the outbreath
- and the pause at the bottom, and also

- the whole of the in breath
- the whole of the next out breath – and so on.

At other times, you can explore a quality, such as texture, or rhythm, depth or sound of the breath. It does not matter what you choose, as long as it engages your interest and helps you move up close to the breath.

There are metaphors we can use – such as 'surfing the waves of the breath' – and 'resting on the breath'. There are phrases that you can repeat silently to yourself – such as 'breath, breathing in', 'breath, breathing out'.

It is helpful to find creative ways of being with the breath – so that you have some favourite tools and approaches that enable you to befriend and attend to the detailed process of breathing.

Difficulties with the breath

There are times when the breath presents us with challenges. Sometimes the breath seems to change as we bring attention to it. It may be that treatment or some association with the breath has influenced this. Perhaps there is no obvious reason, yet a pattern of stilted, tight, or constrained breathing sets in. Practicing with patience and kindly attention may ease things – without trying to change it deliberately, as this may make it worse. It is not unusual, and many of us have times when the breath does not flow as it used to.

If this becomes a regular pattern, the best option may be to find an experienced mindfulness-based teacher. Some one-to-one support, even over the phone or via Skype®, may offer the support that you need.

I offer a few ideas for responding to breathing difficulties here. However, each of us has our own pattern of breathing, so my comments may not be right for you.

'Over breathing'

Sometimes it can feel as if we are running out of breath. The chest gets tighter as each successive in-breath is taken. If this sounds familiar, you might see if it helps to gently 'lean' on the outbreath. It is important not to force things, so gentleness is key here.

> *Allowing the in-breath to come in when it is ready, pausing naturally at the top, and then very gently 'leaning' on the outbreath as it goes out. Then repeating this ... ...*

Continuing to do this, whilst giving attention to the sensations of breathing out, until quite naturally, you may find that the flow of the breath returns. This pattern may return from time to time, and when it does, simply resume the gentle 'leaning' on the outbreath.

Locating the breath

I have encouraged you to attend to the breath deep in the body, if possible – perhaps right into the belly; or maybe somewhere in the chest; or perhaps someplace between the two.

Some of you will have learnt to follow the breath just under the nostrils. This is a good place for cultivating concentrated one pointed attention, but in the approach we are following, it is generally more helpful to come deeper into the body. When attending to the breath at the nostrils, it is as if much of the body, including the trunk, is left out – with all the attention focused up in the head. Thoughts can appear to be perilously close at times.

Coming to the breath down in the body will naturally cultivate a stronger connection with embodied experience, hence the encouragement to attend to the breath there.

If this is not right for you – ignore these suggestions – or experiment with a different focus at different times.

Lack of sensations in the body

Sometimes, it can be difficult to find detailed breath sensations in any of the suggested places. There may be a strong urge to avoid a part of the body that the breath seems to move through – or there may be not much appreciable sensation to connect with. Is it possible to approach any of these issues as an opportunity to be creative and patient? Here are some ideas to experiment with:

1   Finger breathing[8]
Trace the in and out movement of the breath on the fingers. Taking the index finger of your dominant hand, and place it at the base of the thumb of the other hand - moving it up the side of the thumb as you breath in, pausing at the tip of the thumb at the end of the in breath, and then going down the other side of the thumb as you breathe out. Then repeating this in the same way with the rest of the fingers, going up the side as you breathe in, and going down the other side as you breathe out. When you run out of fingers – you just reverse the tracing process from the little finger back to the thumb. Seeing if you can let the movements of your finger mirror the movement of the breath – so that the breath determines the speed of your finger.

2   Hand on belly breathing
Placing your hand on the belly, and feeling the movement of the breath in the belly, beneath your hand. The warmth of your hand helps to keep your attention just at the place where your hand rests and on the movements of the breath beneath.

3   Two places to rest the attention
I once taught mindfulness to an anaesthetist, who knew all about the breath. He placed his attention either side of the ribs and the intercostal muscles that run between them. These muscles provide the mechanical means that move the chest wall, which then facilitates the movement of the breath in and out of the body.

4   Counting the Breath
There are lots of possibilities for counting the breath. Schoolchildren have been taught to breathe with 7/11 s[9] *– count for 7 as you breathe in – and for 11 as you breathe out.*

You can also count full breaths – in/out 1, in/out 2, and so on up to 5 and then start again at 1. If you get lost, go back to the beginning again.

Finding your own way of being creative with the breath is the best possible option. The breath is our ally in bringing mindfulness into everyday life – always there, always different, and always responsive to whatever is going on. When we are calm, the breath tends to have an easier flow. When we are agitated or anxious, the breath tends to get tighter, faster and more constricted. When excited, the breath has another texture and pace – and so on.

'Breathing in, I calm my body.
Breathing out, I smile.
Dwelling in the present moment
I know this is a wonderful moment',

Thich Nhat Hahn[10]

These are the words of Vietnamese monk, Thich Nhat Hahn. He invites us to repeat these phrases to ourselves as we breathe, as we are present with the breath.

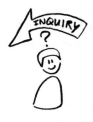

Short Practice Review

1. **The Body Barometer**
2. **A Simple Breathing Space**

Generating your own questions about what you are noticing from the practices you followed last month. Or, using ones we have followed before, to reflect internally on:

What is new in my learning since starting these two practices?
What do they offer?
What am I discovering about myself, if anything?

Developing inquiry

Mindfulness practice, like much else, can become automatic and goal driven. We are usually orientated to having desired outcomes in mind. Applied to mindfulness, this risks turning it into mere 'technique'. By cultivating curiosity and being open to learn from your experience, whatever that is (pleasant or unpleasant), you are nurturing the potential for cultivating compassion and insight throughout your life, and not just limited to your practice.

A Short Inquiry Process that further develops your learning from practice. There are three layers of inquiry[11] and these are explored immediately after, or perhaps even during the practice:

1   What were some *direct experiences* of that practice? What sensations did I notice in the body? What was the 'weather' of the mind? (such as; mood, emotional feelings, thoughts, wandering mind, etc.) and did this change?
2   *How was that?* (How was it to have these experiences? Pleasant or unpleasant?)
3   Is there any *new understanding* that I can draw from this? (for example, things change; noticing difference between being in automatic and coming back to be present; being more kindly towards wandering mind, pushing away the unpleasant, etc.)

You can use this inquiry process after any of your practices.

Recognizing personal patterns

We covered this in some detail in Chapter 3.

Have you had any thoughts or reflections on your own patterns?
What strategies are you developing?
What responses are you finding helpful?

Unpleasant Experience Exercise

You were invited to pay special attention to some unpleasant experiences over the last month, so that in learning more about the way we tend to react to them, we can respond to them more skilfully. We used 'the Blob' once more to map them.

What did you discover?
Did you notice any resistance to exploring the unpleasant?
How did you get on with using the Blob?

Here is an example of an unpleasant experience. Tanya was on her way to clinic for a check-up. She was already a bit late, but then she took a wrong turn, which made her very late. Notice the different layers of her experience.

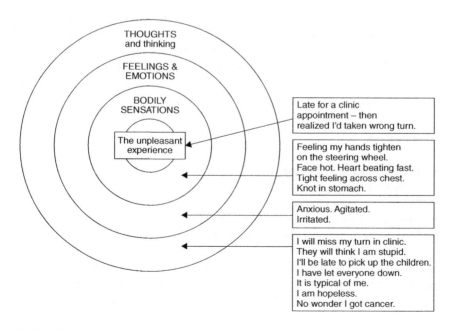

It all happens so fast. We take a wrong turn, which is such an everyday occurrence – and in come a torrent of thoughts, including some nasty judgements. These are quickly followed by uncomfortable feelings, which can build into intense emotions. The whole experience can result in considerable suffering and distress.

Let us slow it all down and see what is happening.

We assumed in the description above that the thoughts came first, but as we discovered earlier (in Walking Down the Street exercise *page 89*), we are often not aware of the part thoughts play in the process. We tend to notice feelings more readily.

The body is highly sensitive to events. If we could separate the dimensions of experience as they happen, we may find that physical sensations show up first for many of us. The body often reacts to very early signs of stress, long before the mind gets in on the act. However, we are often not aware of this.

Thoughts are nothing like as reliable as we believe them to be. They are greatly influenced by prevailing mood or mind state. In this instance, Tanya was on her way to a follow-up clinic. We might assume that she was already feeling anxious. An unpleasant experience (the wrong turn and consequently being late) resulted in further reactivity (catastrophic thoughts and negative judgements), thereby fuelling the intensity of the emotions and the whole experience. Yet we rarely question our thoughts or learn to take current mood into account.

A group of mindfulness participants were discussing the way that thoughts can 'feed' an unpleasant experience. One of the men said that he tended to get angry and move into 'fight' mode. Someone in the group noticed that there were a number of 'F' words, which add to the unpleasant.

Here they are:

- Feed or Fuel (e.g. catastrophic thoughts)
- Fight (e.g. getting angry, blaming)
- Flight (e.g. running away, avoiding)
- Freeze (e.g. unable to take action, ignoring)
- Fix (e.g. trying to solve a situation inappropriately)

These all describe ways that we inadvertently add 'extra' to unpleasant experiences – yet are typical of how we react. Thoughts are always involved in building these 'F' words. They hold the potential of turning an experience that is

ordinarily unpleasant, into something that has the potential to flood and overwhelm. This kind of experience does not just impact at the time, but can linger
for some days or longer, especially if we are unaware of how it built. The
storyline that fuelled it in the first place, may repeat over and over – becoming
more and more convincing. This causes deep suffering.

What can we do?
How can we be with unpleasant experiences differently?

> Diana found some worrying symptoms and was waiting for test results.
> Understandably, she felt anxious during the 10 day wait. By keeping
> physically occupied and doing the Body Scan every day, she managed
> her state of mind reasonably well. However, after coffee out with a
> friend, she felt very panicky and upset. 'She is such a good friend', Diana
> explained. 'I know she was trying to help. But tempting as it is, to go
> over all the possibilities – it actually just made things a lot worse.'

Here are some ideas for reducing the risk of unpleasant experiences growing
into something worse:

- Follow a favourite practice to help you build momentum in Coming Back
  to present moment experience.
- Pay particular attention to the Body Barometer.
- Form an intention to follow a short practice regularly and frequently (even
  if for just a few moments).
- Notice the temptation of moving to add an 'F' word that continues the
  'story' and reinforces the judgements.
- Remember that thoughts are not facts (and now read on!).

Working With Thoughts And Thinking

Let us develop this focus on thoughts and thinking a bit further. It would be helpful to learn to distinguish between thoughts that skilfully clarify a situation for us and those that unhelpfully add extra to what may already be difficult (such as with the F words above). Thoughts are often interpretations of events rather than some firm reality – yet it is so easy to get caught in loops of negative thinking, especially at times of stress and challenge. Learning to relate to thoughts differently can bring some remarkable benefits.

The Sea Of Reactions (Part Two)

We will now link back to an exercise from the previous chapter. In the first part of the Sea of Reactions, you drew out words that described the unhelpful ways that you can react when your buttons are pressed.

If you used your notebook for this, you can refer back to it. If not, choose one word from the list below, or add your own, that for you represents a typical reaction to being stressed or under pressure – something that you know is not helpful.

withdraw	angry	isolated
anxious	irritated	sleep
rush	judge	blame
drink	panic	agitated
eat chocolate	can't sleep	blame

Having chosen your word, write it down on a piece of paper and add thoughts around it that might go with this word.

I have written an example below to help you see what to do.
My original word:

ANXIOUS

Thoughts that I might add to this:

What if everything goes wrong?
If that happens, I'm not sure I'll be able to cope.

Other people manage this much better than I do.
How stupid to keep reacting like this.
I am stupid.

Thoughts often come in groups or linked in threads. One thought leads to another, and then another. Notice in the example that the first thought was making things bigger – expanding possibilities – suggesting a catastrophe. 'What if' and 'everything' are key warning signs. The second thought made future assumptions. If this happens, that will happen. Then the next thought moved into comparing mind (other people …) with negative judgement (manage much better than I do) and the next moves to a global and unkind judgement (How stupid to keep reacting like this!). The final thought identifies the thinker as stupid, as if it was an obvious conclusion to draw.

Patterns of thoughts like these clearly make things worse, yet we keep reacting in this way – and this tends to lower mood, and add extra on top of wherever we started – in this case, heightening anxiety.

One approach[12] is to look at thoughts that feed distress, and ask:

Is this thought necessarily true?
What is the evidence for and against the truth of this thought?
Is there another thought that might be more valid?

We automatically assume that thoughts have validity. If I think this, it must be the case. It can help to question these assumptions.

Let us look at thoughts in another way that might clarify this further.

A seed of reality

When you read the lines below, pause at the end of each line and see what you understand. Do any images come to mind? What do you make of it?

John was on his way to school

He was worried about the maths lesson

He was not sure he could control the class again today

It was not part of a caretaker's duty.

You probably found that your picture of John changed as you read the different lines. At the beginning, you may have seen him as a little lad, perhaps in shorts with a schoolbag. Then he begins to get older as we imagine him worrying about his maths lesson. In the third line, perhaps he became a teacher – and finally, we hear that he is a janitor, or a caretaker. So in a short time, he has aged from under 10, to maybe quite old!

What do you make of this?

It demonstrates the way we interpret pieces of information. The mind is always trying to make meaning out of the information it has to hand. This capacity is so helpful in many ways. It allows us to process and make sense of information, which helps us to navigate many of the complexities of the world we live in.

However the same faculty can also mislead us – as we often draw conclusions that are based on very little material. Images quickly form in the mind and meaning then follows. As we get more information, we update both the meaning and the images that we are seeing – but we do not realize that this is what we are doing. We are unaware of the process that enables us to draw conclusions. We think that we simply see it as it is. There is a seed of reality (John is on his way to school) and all the rest is our interpretation.

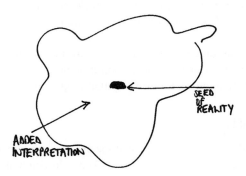

Let us apply this to a familiar context – such as Peter having his bloods taken. The Seed of Reality is:

Last time Peter had bloods taken by a particular nurse, it was painful and took a long time.

The Interpretation around the seed is:

'If she does it again, I will be black and blue, it will hurt a lot, and be as bad as last time.'

'She is no good at her job and should not be allowed to take bloods.'
'I am a coward to hate this as much as I do.'

We can see from this example that the interpretations we make of the event is strongly influenced by what we bring to it. Peter was dreading having bloods taken. He was stuck in the past and what happened last time – and convinced that the same thing would happen again if the same nurse took blood from him. From there he moved into blaming the nurse and judging himself. Yet he does not know what will happen this time.

THOUGHTS ARE NOT FACTS
(Even The Ones That Say That They Are)

Moods and emotions shape the way we see the world. This in turn influences our interpretations. If Peter had been feeling generally optimistic, his frame of mind would be different. As it was, he was dreading the experience, even before he arrived, and this contributed a lot to the way he interpreted what was likely to happen. Feelings – optimistic or dreading – lead to the way our thoughts unfold – positive or negative. This close link between thoughts and feelings results in making thoughts seem very real. It is hard to see thoughts as thoughts – as a vicious cycle can easily get set up that keeps things stuck and seemingly entrenched.

'I always have a bad time having bloods taken.'

If we can see thoughts as events in the mind, we are less likely to be swept away by them. Viewing thoughts like the weather of the mind – always changing, sometimes pleasant, sometimes difficult – is a way to relate to them differently. The art lies in recognizing thoughts as thoughts – remembering that like much else, they come and go. We learn this within the sitting practice and can bring this into everyday life.

The Body Barometer is our ally here – alerting us to upcoming 'weather' and offering a window in which we can interrupt the flow of thoughts, and respond skilfully. We can choose what to do next, rather than be swept away by the rush of thinking.

Kindness is another key, knowing that even the distress connected to a convincing storyline comes and goes – and every moment is an opportunity to start again, come back, touch the bead on your wrist, and be gentle with yourself and your habits of mind.

Relating to thoughts summary

- Seeing thoughts as events in the mind, coming and going, like passing weather.
- Remember that thoughts are not facts – even those that say they are.
- Coming Back to the body and the breath – as ways of staying present.
- Is there any evidence for this thought? Or is it an interpretation of the mind?
- Recognizing the trigger of unpleasant events, and catching the 'F' words.
- Using the Body Barometer to notice signs of stress and pressure.

Buffalo

Still they come, my thoughts
Trampling like a herd of buffalo
Through the green prairie of my mind
Leaving their black footprints in the smooth pasture.

But I am Mountain Man.
They do not scare me now
And I watch them moving by
With no more than passing interest.

Geraint

The Experience Of Cancer

Living With Cancer

Wellness And Illness

Many more people now live longer with cancer. As treatment outcomes improve, and clinical research offers more understanding, cancer can become a long-term condition. Surviving cancer may mean the need for continuous or frequent treatments. This has personal costs as well as benefits. Advances in treatment extend lives, but the regimes invariably have an impact.

This book is dedicated to helping you find some tools and resources that might help, however your life and health is at this time. All the approaches in this book are offered to support you wherever you are in the path of wellness and illness. Use whichever support you best.

Making the most of the time that is left

Some people are fortunate to find they feel stronger each year post-treatment. For them, in time, the experience of cancer begins to fade. It perhaps no longer takes up the central ground it once did. At first, cancer seems to identify us. It becomes the lens through which we view the world – and the way the world seems to see us. Yet we are so much more than our cancer.

I remember someone challenging my use of the term 'people with cancer'. She told me that whilst she acknowledged that she had been diagnosed with cancer in the past, she no longer had it – so she was not 'someone with cancer' now. However, even after several years have slipped by, anxiety can still return, especially around check-up times. The shadow of cancer tends to linger on some occasions, such as anniversaries.

Those who stay well after treatment are the lucky ones. You are among the many whose lives have been saved by advances in treatment, care and research. To you and all others, who may be less fortunate, this question seems important:

How can you use this experience of cancer to make the most of your life?

> After treatment for breast cancer, Chris felt strongly that she wanted to 'make a difference' in some way. Once she was well enough, she went out to work in an East European orphanage for a few weeks.

> Joe was determined to get fit again after his treatment. He embarked on a series of sponsored walks to raise money for a national cancer charity.

> Ben had always wanted to develop his writing. He started a blog for men with the same rare cancer as he had. He found it rewarding when someone made a comment about how much his blog was helping.

All these people and many others like them find some way to make the most of their lives after cancer. The rest of us can too, by enjoying and finding meaning in activities that have personal significance.

> Beryl goes into her garden every day. 'In the old days', she told me, 'I would go out and long for a favourite flower to come into bloom – not really noticing what was there in front of me. Now I go deliberately to see what is there.'

> Joanna has incurable cancer. She spends a lot of time with her five grand-
> children – teaching them to bake, helping with homework, babysitting,
> and hearing about their days. 'Before I got cancer, I was busy working. I
> didn't have much spare time', she said. 'I am strangely happier now than
> I have ever been, even though I don't know how long I have.'

Can we allow the experience of life-threatening illness to help us make the
most of each day? Can the shock of this illness wake us up to the life we are
living now? This calls on us to be more kind and less judging to those moments
that challenge us; to be present to the detail of the beauty that surrounds us; and
to appreciate the people and the activities that we care about.

This ageing, changing body

Many of us are living with some level of chronic condition, perhaps as a result
of treatment, and maybe due to the inevitable wear and tear of passing years.
This may involve some lasting disability. There may be grief and a sense of loss
over what once was, and is no longer. How to be present with what is here now?

Perhaps there is pain, less energy, reduced sleep, food we can no longer
tolerate, psychological challenges, poorer concentration, and changed body
image and strength. These are all things that can limit us and can loom large at
times. How might we fold them into the inevitability of this body changing,
getting ill and ageing? How can we be present with what is here now?

How to use mindfulness practice to live
– *as fully as we can;*
– *as happily as we are able, and*
– *as kindly to ourselves and the world as is possible?*

Responding to difficulty

There are every day challenges and life events for each of us at times, whatever
our current health status. Difficulties may come from cancer, from something
quite different, or from a variety of sources. Whatever the cause, what matters
is how we respond to it.

At the start of this book, we explored the possibility that it is not so much the
difficulty itself that causes our suffering – but the way we relate to it.

What do you make of this statement now? Does it confuse or irritate as it may
once have done? I wonder if the mindfulness practice that you have developed,

and the life experiences that you have grown through, help you to have more insight into what this implies?

Through my work with people with cancer, I notice that it is not necessarily those with the most intense challenges who suffer the most. Sometimes the person with the best prognosis in a roomful of people with cancer is the most anxious. He or she is not wrong to feel like that. That could be any one of us. There are so many factors influencing mood, emotion and reactivity. Being at the mercy of anxiety is very distressing – yet little by little, we can cultivate the means to relate more gently to what challenges us. This is not a linear development. We are bound to find that mood and reactivity change, even within a day. However, when we discover ways of putting learning into practice, responding kindly, then experience itself starts to transform and our understanding with it.

Claudia had to go for check-ups at least every three months. She had bladder cancer, and had had several local recurrences. She dreaded the whole experience and tended to become distressed, even as she walked across the threshold of the clinic. Greatly to her and her nurses' surprize, on one occasion she breathed through the procedure. She stayed calm all the way through. Later appointments were not always as markedly successful, but Claudia saw clearly after that first time, that how she reacted made a big difference to her experience of these times. From then on, she always used her breath to support her.

Recurrence

A recurrence of cancer is what we all dread. You may have gone through treatment and feel more or less recovered. Life has returned to near normal – although both psychologically and physically, you may be different now to how you were before you were first diagnosed. Enough time may have passed that thoughts of possible recurrence have faded somewhat.

We think of the past as solid, unchangeable and fixed – but in hindsight, things can develop differently to how they appear at the time. This may be the case when we first heard about a recurrence. It does not mean that everything turns out fine, but perhaps something that appears to be very difficult and fixed, may not prove to be quite so serious in time. Experiencing a recurrence is bound to be disappointing at best, and shattering at worst. It may prove to be somewhere between the two.

Diagnosis tools – what helps?

This time of recurrence may appear similar to how it was when you were first diagnosed. You may feel shocked and shaky. You may feel angry and enraged. It may be a sense of deep grief that affects you the most. Whatever you feel, let yourself express it – to friends, family, health professionals or even to the tree at the bottom of the garden, or at the top of the hill, where few people go.

Since your original diagnosis, you have had the experience of managing all sorts of physical and psychological challenges, finding sources of trustworthy information and developing comprehensive knowledge of the medical system and what is on offer. You have learnt a lot about negotiating the territory and hopefully you have had people and resources available to support you.

It may be worth sitting down with your notebook at some point and listing the resources that have helped you since you were first diagnosed – especially:

- the things that nurtured you
- the things you did that helped
- the people and places who are there to support you (are they the same or different to who were there for you at the beginning?)
- the mindfulness approaches that you carry with you
- the mindfulness core practices that may be most helpful.

Noticing the stories, spinning in the mind

Now is the chance to use the learning we have been exploring around thoughts, emotions and interpretations. It might be helpful to keep checking whether your ideas about your current situation are well founded.

You might draw a picture of the seed of reality (the clear facts around the recurrence) and the bigger area of interpretation surrounding (your internal stories, unchecked information, current medical guesswork, etc.)

Keep coming back to what you definitely know. Prognoses change – often improving from what was first thought, and yes, sometimes getting worse.

Resilience

We are often not aware of the many ways that we change through experience. We assume certain constant qualities and characteristics, but this denies all the myriad experiences that shape us from day-to-day and year-to-year. Treatment and diagnosis may have made their mark and while you are bound to have some negative memories of that time, perhaps these experiences have also offered you rich learning and many opportunities for growing and changing.

The term 'resilience' is linked to the physical properties of something such as steel, which is made strong by combining different metals and tempering them at very high temperatures. As a result, steel has the ability to stay intact under extreme conditions. Psychological resilience is the capacity of the individual to cope with change. Here are some of the factors that are found in people who have developed resilience, in the context of coping with intense difficulty.[13]

1   Being able to make a realistic plan and having the ability to see it through.
2   Having a generally positive attitude towards ones strengths and abilities.
3   Having communication and problem solving skills.
4   Ability to manage strong impulses and emotions.

Those of us who have navigated treatment and diagnosis have been 'tempered' like steel. There are complex factors behind the way that we individually respond to difficult times, but research suggests that many of us thrive and grow despite the adverse conditions we go through.[14]

Inviting you to review this for yourself internally or in your notebook:

In what ways have I changed since being diagnosed?
In what ways am I stronger?
What have I learnt about myself, and about life?
In view of everything that has happened, what really matters to me now?

Intention

> *Once you have reflected on these questions in your own way – you might go to sit in a favourite place, inside or out, with your feet firmly on the ground - and coming to the breath, bringing attention to your breathing in your own way for a few minutes.*
>
> *Once you feel ready, turning to your intention for the next few weeks. Depending on the context, and the challenges that you have ahead of you, cultivating once more an overarching intention that speaks to what you most need – that points you in the direction of what will serve you best. As you sit and breathe, forming your intention, remember to breath into your heart, and calling on the innate wisdom of the heart to guide you.*

At the end of this practice, you might want to record your intentions in your journal – perhaps making a list of how these might be translated into everyday activities and practices that will support you.

The Thread Exercises

 Whatever level of wellness or illness you might be experiencing, these next three exercises link directly with the thread and bring together a number of practices that you have been developing. The first is Feet on the Floor; the second is the same as Coming to the Breath, focusing attention on the belly; and the third connects you with Kindness and others who are practicing with the threads. You can practice them separately or together – and ideally you need a thread to help you follow this practice.

---

1   Feet on the Floor ... ... Exploring

Putting the mind and attention into feeling the Feet on the Floor and exploring all the detailed sensations in toes, and balls of the feet, and heels. Noticing texture, contact, pressure, pain (if there is any), ease, weight, sensation and so on. Doing this for a few moments several times a day – maybe when we link to a daily activity (such as getting up from bed, or finished eating). When awake in bed at night – then putting the mind and attention into the contact of the body with the bed or floor.

2   Hand on the belly... ... ... Breathing

Placing the hand on the belly and inviting the mind to move to the breath moving under the hand. Feeling the sensations of the belly moving and noticing how the hand moves with the belly as we breathe in and breathe out. Doing this for a little while several times a day – noticing when the mind wanders to something else (which is quite normal and not a problem) – and seeing if it is possible to gently come back to the breath and the belly and the hand. This is a helpful thing to do whenever we are stressed, or under pressure. Just stopping what we are doing and turning to the breath can help us to notice what is happening and then choose what to do next.

3   Touching the bead... ... ... Connecting

Touching the bead, linking into the heart and opening to the possibility of sending kindness to ourselves. Not forcing this, just opening to the

---

possibility. Coming to the Breath with Kindness. Repeating one of these phrases if you would like, or adapting your own:

May I be safe and protected, in the midst of change and uncertainty.
May I be peaceful in the midst of fear.
May I live with kindness.

You can also touch the bead, linking again into the heart and thinking of others who are ill or having tough times and wishing them well wherever they are. Many people are wearing threads. Many have cancer. It is best to do this exercise for yourself first before moving on to do it for others.

Nicole was on holiday in South America, celebrating a significant birthday. Unfortunately, she developed altitude sickness, which seriously affected her breathing. On her way to hospital for treatment, while travelling on a local bus, things got a lot worse. 'I felt quite alone', she told me. 'I was really struggling for breath and feeling very anxious. I don't know why I remembered, but I reached over and found the bead on my thread. It was quite remarkable. I thought of all the other people who might be struggling for breath or feeling alone – and this helped me to relax, which eased my breathing a lot.'

Intention For The 'Month' Of Kindness

Take as long as you want to work through this chapter – doing it in whatever way serves you best. There is no advantage in covering the ground quickly. Savouring your moments is itself an act of kindness.

Here are the practices for you to follow. All of them are available to download, see the Companion website at the front of this book for more information.

Practices – for this 'month'

Core Practice
— Walking with Kindness [10 + a fortnight/20 + a month]
Alternating with another core practice if you want

Short Practices
— Coming to the Breath with Kindness [daily]
— 3 Step Responding Space – [2 or 3 × a day]
Continuing with other short practices of your choice

Cancer Practice – with the thread

The Three Thread Exercises   – *whenever you need them*
— Feet on the Floor – Exploring
— Hand on the Belly – Breathing
— Touching the Bead – Connecting

You will have noticed that all of the practices build on what has gone before. By now, you may have your own adaptations and ways of practicing. This is a helpful development. By making them your own, you will be weaving them into your day.

Intention

However, your intention remains important. As mindfulness practice becomes more integrated into your day, habits of forgetfulness can still slip in. Practice itself risks becoming automatic and old habits may return. By staying creative and curious, keeping your practice fresh and new, you remember why this is important:

What really matters to you?
How are you bringing that into everyday reality?

You may not manage all the practices every day, but being willing to find ways to remember, and start over, again and again is our ongoing skilful intention. Be sure to appreciate your efforts. Day-by-day, step-by-step, moment-by-moment is how we bring the beam of mindfulness to nurture our lives.

We try to construct a life in which we will be perfect, in which we will eliminate awkwardness, pass by vulnerability, ignore ineptness, only to pass through the gate of our mind and find, strangely, that the gateway is vulnerability itself. The very place (... where) we are open to the world whether we like it or not.
David Whyte

Notes

1   Christina Feldman talk on 17th September 2014. Available at: www.dharmaseed. org
2   Bates, T. (2005)
3   Rogers, C.R. (1974)
4   Ali Smith interview, Guardian Saturday, Review 5 September 2014, see Clark, A. (2014, September 06)
5   Chödrön, P. (1997)
6   This is adapted from Segal, Williams & Teasdale (2013)
7   This is adapted from Segal, Williams & Teasdale (2013)
8   With thanks to Mindfulness in Schools Project and.b for this approach, see https:// mindfulnessinschools.org/
9   https://mindfulnessinschools.org/
10 Hahn, T.N. (2005)
11 Three layers of inquiry have been developed by teachers from the Centre for Mindfulness, Research and Practice (CMRP), Bangor University, Wales.
12 This approach is from Cognitive Behavior Therapy (CBT) – distraction to reduce the frequency of depressing thoughts (Beck et al., 1979).
13 Fredrickson, B.L. & Branigan, C (2005)
14 Calhoun, L.G. & Tedeschi, R.G. (Eds) (2006, 2014)

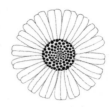

Personal Story

JANE

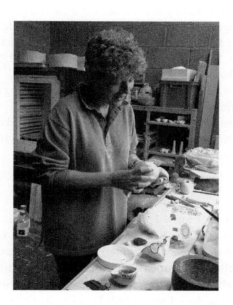

Jane is 49, married, with two children in their 20s. She has lived near the sea all her life and now lives in the house she grew up in, right beside the beach. She started as a pencil artist, then turned to oils and finally came home to ceramics. Her son Michael lives at home. He has a very rare form of cancer and has needed full time care for five years. Jane is his principal carer. She attended a mindfulness course about four years ago and then another three years later.

Mindfulness: A Kindly Approach to Being with Cancer, First Edition. Trish Bartley.
© 2017 John Wiley & Sons, Ltd. Published 2017 by John Wiley & Sons, Ltd.
Companion Website: www.wiley.com/go/bartley/mindfulness

When Michael came home from hospital four years ago, our anaesthetist recommended mindfulness to me. I had previously had counselling.

Michael was 13 when first diagnosed with Von Hippel-Lindau syndrome. That was 13 years ago. It is a very rare form of cancer and he has needed surgery every 18 months or so to remove tumours in his brain and spine. He has been in and out of hospital, many times since being diagnosed.

From the beginning, there was a lot to manage. I did my best to take as much as possible from Michael, so that he could be the 13-year-old that he needed to be. After three years or so, I started to struggle. The worst times were the pauses of normality between surgery.

I worked at the children's school as a nursery assistant and art teacher. If I went into the little ones class, feeling rubbish, I would suddenly find I had a 3-year-old wrapped around my leg, greeting me with 'Hello, Mrs. S'! You could put everything behind you for a bit, but then you go home and it would all crash back in again. It was like a great big turmoil inside, trying to bubble over, but whenever anyone came in, it was squashed. After a time you can only squash so much in. It is like your whole insides are agitated. Your thoughts are agitated. I had to keep busy to satisfy that agitation.

I could get off to sleep, but if I woke up, I would be going through things in my head, like sorting a filing cabinet. I might say to myself, 'I'm not going to think about Michael' and then all sorts of other things would crowd in – a child at school, something I need to do … Things got faster at night – so I would get up and go and do something to stop the thoughts.

Getting help

I got to a point where I knew I wasn't coping. I would go to my GP for no reason, other than to tell him how Michael was. I couldn't keep still. My feet and hands were on the move all the time. He suggested I talk to someone, so I went to a counsellor. We formed a nice relationship. She told me that at first I was able to talk about everything and anything except myself. Whenever she asked me how I was feeling, I just clamped up. I couldn't speak. It was literally as if someone was holding me here (*pointing to her neck*).

She knew my love of art and suggested that I just draw – not think about it – but take a pencil and just draw what was happening. When I showed it to her, she said she had never seen so much on one piece of paper. Everything was on it. She used the picture to start me talking. That was about 10 years ago. My drawing developed into writing and that was when I started writing poetry. I filled ten or so books.

There were other family issues to deal with as well as Michael. Eventually things got so bad that P, my husband, insisted that we go away for a week without a phone. His parents looked after the children and we had a week away just the two of us. I'll never forget it. It was one of those very special times. Everything had a meaning. I believe there was an element in that holiday that I've looked for ever since. It was vital to have that time as a couple. P knew that.

In December 2007, P had surgery to his hip and the next summer, Michael needed several lots of surgery and radiotherapy. It was such a long year. Finally, he had surgery to a tumour that was wrapped around the brain stem. That took everything from Michael – his ability to breathe whilst asleep, to feed himself, to talk (he had a tracheostomy), and to walk. He had been living independently and had completed the second year of his architectural degree. That all stopped.

We had the garage converted into high dependency for Michael. We had a sense of what was in store. We fortunately had a lot of help from a cancer charity for children and young people (CLIC Sargent [www.clicsargent.org.uk]). We just managed to get it finished in time for Michael to come home for Christmas 2009.

Mindfulness

The anaesthetist who helped get Michael home, picked up on how I was. I was back to moving a lot, couldn't sit still and she suggested I might try mindfulness.

When I met you (Trish), you taught me three mindfulness exercises and gave me a thread to help remember to do them. I tried the Feet on the Floor on the beach and it made me enjoy the beach all the more. I used it in bed, by feeling the duvet over my feet. That helped when I woke at night. I would go back to sleep, by feeling the duvet over my toes and follow it up my legs. I don't think I ever got further than my knees.

I remember thinking 'these are working' – but life still carried on relentlessly. I was driving back and forward to Liverpool every day for 10 months, before Michael came home. It was all a bit crazy. When I first met you, we talked about the course and I really didn't think I could manage 'turning towards' the difficult. It felt too much. But I needed a window of peace – you know, that moment when everything falls away. That was what got me to mindfulness. I had a taste of it on the beach and in the bed – so it was 'ok, lets try. I must do something'.

I found the course really hard the first time. I struggled to find the time for me. The Body Scan was long. My brain couldn't hang on for that length of time, let alone my body. That's why I stuck with the pause and the feet on the floor, because they were instant. I liked the little coloured sticky dots. I had one on my car keys – others on the fridge door, laptop, and one on my spice drawers. If they caught my eye, in that split second, there was a recognition of 'Yes, stop!'. It was like someone saying 'Wake up', 'Don't go down that road again.' You can tell yourself, 'It's okay. Nothing bad will happen if you stop'. That was the first time I'd had something as visual. Automatic pilot was most definitely my way of life – especially with all the driving I was doing.

From that first course, I learnt to stop, to pause, and to get my feet on the floor – little tiny interruptions. The agitation declined with that ability to stop. Does that make sense? There wasn't the need to keep going, because I could interrupt things. Also Michael was starting to do well. We still had the odd battle to get things in place – but he was home. We had done it! We'd got him back.

Second mindfulness course

By Nov 2012, Michael had had the longest gap ever between surgery since he was first diagnosed. We had been watching a tumour on the brain stem and knew there was another on the spine. Michael started to struggle a bit. It was very high-risk to operate on the brain stem. We had a fair idea where things were going.

It was at that point that you just start to think – I'm heading back down that road again. I know where I am going. And instead of allowing it to start, I thought, 'I'm going to have to get back into mindfulness again'. So I wrote to you.

I had lost a lot of my support people. For anyone in my shoes I would say, 'Keep talking. Don't go inward too much. Talk to someone who is trained to listen'. If you want to look after someone, you must care for yourself. I'm not very good at talking to friends. I knew that if I took a mindfulness course again, I had to give it my commitment. That lack of compromise was helpful. If I had been left with some wriggle room – 'come when you can' – I probably wouldn't have made it. There is always a reason not to come.

I had a lot of trouble practicing mindfulness in the house when I was doing the second course. So I would go and practice with the CD player in the car. When I am in the house trying to practice, I am constantly on guard listening. Taking myself away is almost a preparation for being able to move into practice.

Now I often go and walk on the beach. I stand with no shoes on, feeling the water lapping against my feet. I can feel my feet going into the sand. You know how they disappear? That's a lovely feeling.

P, my husband, is a bit sceptical about mindfulness, although he supports me to do whatever will help. His way is through sailing. When he is in the water, he says he cannot focus on anything else. 'That is what mindfulness is!' I told him. My ceramics is like P's sailing. I have a little studio, directly opposite Michael. It is out of the actual house, but I can see straight into his room when the crab apple tree is not in leaf. I am still too close, but I don't want to be too far. You can't work quickly with clay. You have to allow the clay to develop and take form. I feel it – soft – I work it – then it goes leather hard – and then I polish it with a little glass bead – and then I brush it with a fine slip called *terra sigillata*. I make little globes like worry balls.

Mindfulness and Michael

Michael's future now is uncertain. Three weeks ago he was told that surgery is not an option. As a family, we are striving to keep things as normal as possible. He is scared.

Like us all, he will tend to dwell on the things that bother him. He gets all sorts of pictures in his head. 'Will it be like this?'

So I encourage him to focus on where he is now. 'Is it a beautiful day?' 'Yes it is.' 'Can you hear the sparrows in our box hedge?' I use the example of the mind being a bit like a puppy. I say to him, 'Your mind is pulling you down a road that you don't want to go down.' (He adores Molly, our Springer Spaniel). 'Imagine it is Molly pulling down the wrong road. You are not going to let her. Say to her, "lets go this way instead".' I tell him to use this for himself.

When he is wound up and upset, I say to him 'Come on, just stop for a minute. Feel where you are. Just breathe'. I'm trying to bring in things that have helped me. That has a knock-on effect. It helps me and I hope it helps Michael. I don't know if he does this without me, but he certainly does it with me, when he is getting wound up – and it seems to help him.

P and I are trying to put things in place. We have the blue bag ready now, with morphine and the syringe driver and all that – and I need to know what is in it and what needs doing. Every time we discuss it, it is making it real. We have known we would reach this point since his diagnosis. He has had eight brain and two spinal tumours removed – you almost become complacent. And now after all these years, there is nothing more they can do. You wonder, 'Is this actually happening?'

One morning recently, we were walking the dogs on the beach and we met a friend. She always asks how we all are – and how Michael is. I looked at her and I just couldn't speak. 'Not doing so well today?' she asked kindly. And I nodded. The agitation wasn't there – just this knot in my throat, which stops me talking. I feel it a bit now but I can come back to my feet on the floor to steady me.

The floor never changes – it might change texture – but it is there whatever happens with Michael. It is there and a constant. All the people this beach has seen – but the rocks, the boat pool, the sea coming in and the sea going out hasn't changed.

Michael died at home a few months after this interview. Two years later, Jane started a degree in applied arts specializing in ceramics. The personal theme for her work is 'Broken is Beautiful'.

What If?

Two small words
What if?
Two small words
What if?

Mind starts spinning
What if?
Stomach is lurching
What if?

Knots all inside
What if?
Body shaking
What if?

Feeling sick
What if?
Panic grips
What if?

What if?
STOP!
PAUSE!
BREATHE!
FEET ON THE FLOOR!

(take a pause here)

Mind slowing
Knots undoing
Stillness growing
Panic fading

What if?
If what?

Jane

Chapter 5
Completing And Continuing

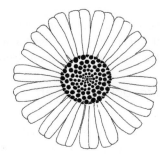

I love all beginnings, despite their uncertainty ... if I wish that something had not happened; if I doubt the worth of an experience and remain in my past – then I choose to begin at this very second.
  Begin what? I begin. I have already just begun a thousand lives.

Rainer Maira Rilke[1]

It may seem a little strange to start this chapter about 'completing' with a quotation about 'beginning'. However, mindfulness is all about cultivating 'beginner's mind' – and this chapter is all about beginning to bring mindfulness into the rest of your life.

Mindfulness: A Kindly Approach to Being with Cancer, First Edition. Trish Bartley.
© 2017 John Wiley & Sons, Ltd. Published 2017 by John Wiley & Sons, Ltd.
Companion Website: www.wiley.com/go/bartley/mindfulness

Completing Thus Far

We often say to mindfulness participants that what matters most is what happens *after* the course has finished. This is true for you too.

The intention is to support your wellbeing, whatever the current state of your health. This may sound like a bit of a contradiction. How can there be 'wellbeing' if you are still receiving treatment for cancer? How can you be 'well' if you often feel anxious about cancer returning? This chapter is dedicated to finding out.

Freedom from fear

If we cultivate a vision that is optimistic – but not fixed on any specific outcome – we may go beyond what we now think is possible. Others have done this before you, by reducing the extremes of their reactivity. 'Mindfulness takes the tops off the waves' was how someone with advanced cancer described it.

In any moment, there is the potential to focus on the pleasant or the unpleasant. We assume that our inner experience is largely determined by external events. A beautiful day brings pleasure and ease. Lingering low flat cloud and wet mist produces claustrophobia and dullness. But we do not have to be at the mercy of events. Things happen – often out of our control. What matters is how we relate to them – in what comes next.

You may have experienced challenges that you never imagined you would have to endure – or be able to withstand. But even in the wildest weather, there is shelter to be found. You can find your way to somewhere safe – when a Body Scan practice helps you find some respite; when a walk through autumn leaves unaccountably lifts your mood – it can feel possible to pick up and start again.

What do you need to put in place to continue responding to both the challenges and opportunities that come into your world?

Integrating practice into the everyday

We first undertake a review in order to evaluate what has been helpful. If you have been using a notebook, now is the time to read back through it.

> Ruth wrote a letter to her mindfulness teacher, explaining that she had moved away from the area. She said that she was sorry to admit that she did very little practice these days. At the end of the letter, she thanked her teacher for helping her at such a difficult time, and said that she didn't know where she would be now without the breath.

This is not an unusual story. Ruth obviously connected mindfulness with the core practices. Coming back to the breath had simply become something she folded into her day.

Over time, we tend to absorb new learning into the fabric of our lives, almost forgetting where it came from. At the beginning, it may feel awkward. After a while, if we persevere, it feels more natural and becomes a habit – a good one, if it is supportive for you.

This is why it is worth reviewing your practice every now and again. We forget things when life improves. Staying in touch with your practice is insurance for what might lie ahead. We naturally hope tough times will never come again. However, life is full of ups and downs, and old patterns readily surface when we are under pressure. If you have developed effective tools and learned to use them skilfully, it is important to keep them in good order, so that they are there when you need them.

Jon Kabat-Zinn's wise advice is often quoted:

> *Weave your parachute every day.*
> *You never know when you might need it.*[2]

Letting this guide you as you decide how to sustain your practice.

Reviewing the four movements

These movements form the practice of mindful awareness As you review your learning, it is good to find ways to remember each of the movements.

Intention

Offers direction and vision. As if following a compass bearing, the cultivation of wise intention keeps you aligned with what really matters. By connecting with this, your intention sustains your practice, guides your choices, and underpins everyday mindful living.

Appreciating the beauty of nature meant a lot to Mary. Friends knew this and would often bring her flowers. Forming an intention to spend time with something beautiful every day, she often stood at the window gazing at the changing details of the shapes, colours, and movements of the plants, trees and flowers – breathing in the beauty of her garden.

Coming back

Is shorthand for the movement of mind that returns to present moment experience. The mind's automatic tendency is to wander off into thoughts, stories and inner commentaries, luring you into believing and following them. Instead, on a good day, you notice and come back to the anchor of the body and the breath – to being grounded in the present.

Mindfulness is the beam of light that illuminates the wandering mind, and shows the way back. Sometimes we focus on detail and sometimes we expand out into a wider landscape.

Oliver was very unwell, but he loved to walk amongst the trees near the river. He knew how much it helped him to stay steady and not get swept away by cascades of anxious thoughts. When he got to the river, he would pause, feeling his feet on the ground. Then he would widen his gaze up the river and take it all in – the flow of the water, the sounds, the movement of the trees along the banks, the air on his skin, his body standing there. 'It is deeply nourishing', he said.

Turning towards

Is the movement that responds to the arising of difficulty, once Coming Back is established. Instead of following a natural tendency to avoid what is unpleasant, or get caught up in the story of the difficulty, we turn towards the felt sense of difficulty in the body. Gently exploring the sensations, using the breath for support – we bring kindness in on the breath to wherever it is felt in the body, allowing it to be there.

Sometimes this seems like a step too far. If there is a risk of feeling overwhelmed or flooded, we wisely find another place to stand – perhaps by doing something physical, or getting involved in a quite different activity. When the flood risk has receded, we come back into the body, and breathe with whatever is there.

A radical way of responding to difficulty is to turn towards the lovely. Not artificially creating a positive, but choosing to notice and appreciate the people and places that you love. The mind aligns itself to what it focuses on. Turning towards what is lovely helps us to appreciate what is there and reduces the tendency to get stuck in rumination that fuels what is difficult.

Annie was in pain and looked pale. She slowly made her way to a chair in the corner. Every now and again, I looked across at her, during the mindfulness group session. I could see that she was following everything we were doing. We talked at the end. 'It was really important for me to come today', she said. 'I was determined to practice alongside everyone else. It is true I am in pain, but it was surprisingly helpful to be still – and breathe with it. It was just like they say – I could surf the waves of the pain. It didn't go away. I'm not even sure that the pain got less. But somehow I could hold it and be with it. It is quite weird really, because the pain is pretty bad at times – yet I feel incredibly still and peaceful.'

Kindness

Is the last movement, yet it has been there all along. It is the quality of gentleness that imbues practice and everyday life with a gesture of friendliness. It may not come naturally at first. It needs time, practice and courage to cultivate. Kindliness is the way to heal our sorrows and make space for what matters most to us.

Donna had recently heard that the cancer had spread to the back of her head. We talked for a bit and then practiced together. We started with intention, and then established a grounded seated presence – weight going down, height going up, strong back, soft front. Then we came to the breath, and rested there, breathing for a few minutes. Towards the end of the practice, I invited Donna to notice any part of the body that might benefit from some kindly attention – maybe a place of pain, or tenderness.

We talked afterwards and Donna told me that she had turned towards the area where she knew the cancer had spread. She said it was as if she was cupping the area gently in her hands – 'like two measures of tenderness', she said, quoting a favourite poem.[3] And how did this feel?' I asked her. 'I just felt tenderly towards this place, and less 'churny' in my belly. I feel quite calm now.'

It is tempting to imagine that these four people have been practicing for years. But this is not so. The length of their practice ranges from a few weeks to a couple of years. Significantly, what all four share is a diligent intention to practice every day – through frequent short practices, everyday connections and longer periods of core practice (such as 15–20 minutes), several days a week.

They all know the value of practice. *Without* a regular connection to practice, they find they are more reactive. Troubling thoughts have more impact, emotions are more labile, and mood dips more easily. *With* practice, they are more able to hold pain and distress, whether physical or emotional, with a kinder touch. It is not a static picture of course. There are better and worse days, but there is always the possibility of starting again.

Practice as if your life depends on it.[2]

Jon Kabat-Zinn encourages us to discover that life can be lived more fully with the support of practice.

A Practice Review

The chart below shows the key practices that you have learned. Additional practices were also included in the chapters. Practice needs creativity to stay fresh. Adapting things to suit you will help you to deepen and develop your mindfulness practice.

Key Practices	Intention	Coming Back	Turning Towards	Kindness
Core	Body Scan *page 41*	Mindful Walking *page 73*	Sitting Practice *page 133*	Walking with Kindness *page 178*
Short	The Pause *page 37* Feet on the Floor *page 39*	Standing in Mountain *page 81* Coming to the Breath *page 83*	The Body Barometer *page 148* Simple Breathing Space *page 150*	Coming to the Breath with Kindness *page 182* 3 Step Responding Space *page 184*

Cancer Context	Thread Practice	Practice
Diagnosis	First Aid practice *page 51*	Feet on the Floor (FOF)
Waiting	Waiting Practice *page 99*	Pause + FOF
Treatment	Treatment Practice *page 102*	FOF + Coming to the Breath (C to B)
Uncertainty (post treatment)	Simple Breathing Space *page 156*	Pause + FOF + Coming to the Breath (C to B)
Living with Cancer	The Thread Exercises *page 207*	1) FOF 2) C to B 3) Kindness

There is a simple review process that you can use:

+   What is helpful, enjoyable, effective, etc.?
−   What has been hard to integrate, unhelpful, difficult?
?   Gathering this together, what practices will I choose to continue? How will I weave my parachute every day?

Find your own way of doing this – or deciding now when you will turn to this.

Gathering it together

We conclude this review by sharing part of the Three Circle model[4] from Mindfulness-Based Cognitive Therapy for Cancer,[5] the program this book is based on. It shows how the four movements come together to form the practice of mindful awareness. The outside ring may remind you of the rings of the Blob – the different dimensions of experience.

The Circle of Practice

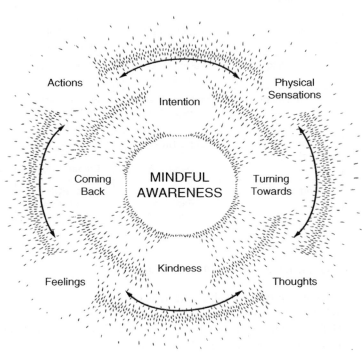

We now form plans and cultivate intentions that will support you to carry on.

Continuing

Daily living

We start by looking at different activities in your day and how they impact on you.

Daily activities diary

1   Make a list of all the things you do, in an ordinary day, from when you wake up, to when you go to bed.
2   Then looking down your list, and categorize each activity using **N** for nourishing, or **D** for draining, or **M** for Mastery. Write **D** or **N** or **M** beside each activity. **N**urturing activities are those that enliven us, and lift the mood. **D**epleting activities are those that drain us, or lower the mood. **M**astery activities are activities like paying bills, cleaning out the fridge, or clearing emails. You may not enjoy doing them at the time, but feel satisfied once they are done.

For example:

- get out of bed   D
- have a shower   N/D
- put the washing on   M
- stand in mountain while the kettle boils   N
- drink a cup of tea   N
- etc.

3   When you have completed your list, reflect on the balance of Ns and Ds in your day.

What makes one activity an N and another a D?
How can I reduce my Ds and increase my Ns?
Are there any Ds that could become Ms?

We often seek enjoyment from things that do not nourish us. Checking the phone every few minutes; shopping online for things not really wanted; going to the fridge and eating, yet not being hungry. There are many ways we try fill the loneliness of an empty space. We long for connection, yet often look in the wrong place.

Much depends on intention and context. I remember a friend watching the whole box set of West Wing over the worst days of his chemotherapy. It gave him a break and felt nourishing.

How can we discern the difference between skilful and unskilful choices? How can we spend more time being fed by life, rather than depleted by it?

Pausing now and again to notice how you are feeling. Deliberately creating a space to come back and ask:

What do I need right now?
How can I best take care of myself?

Balancing different aspects of daily life

Monitoring balance can support self-care and offer a different perspective.

- *Exercise and rest* – do you have enough of each? The immune system replenishes itself when we sleep, so sufficient rest is important. Even if sleep is illusive, using mindfulness to help you rest and give the body time to recharge and heal. Exercise, even if it is quite minimal, enlivens and refreshes the body and the mind. It can lift the mood and walking is excellent mindfulness practice.
- *Having fun and making meaning* – fun and play tend to take a back seat at times of illness, unless you have people round you who are naturally playful. Fun tends to be spontaneous. It is so good for us. Laughter is the best of medicines!

  Making meaning supports resilience. Gaining insight into your own narrative connects you to understanding the universal human condition. We find links with others, who have written, painted, or composed many wonders that enrich what it is to be human.
- *Friends and family* – Illness inevitably limits the scope of social life. Friends may react in unpredictable ways. Some step forward generously; others seem less able to show up. Family and friends are valued sources of support during illness. When life seems more normal, it seems important to pick up on the balance of relationships. Their lives may have been on hold alongside yours – and whilst you may still rely on their support, there may be ways of reaching out to them in kindness and appreciation.
- *Diet and well-being* – the end of treatment is often a time when people review what they eat. There is a wealth of advice available, but it might be wise to take things slowly and gradually. Small sustainable steps are worth

far more then huge changes, quickly dropped. You might add a few healthy ingredients and reduce a few others that are not so good.

There are many potential ways to support well-being. Here are a few ideas:

- enjoying silence
- spending time in nature
- trusting and expressing your feelings
- being creative
- exploring new experiences.

A set of evidence-based actions 'Five ways to well-being'[6] *are used in many* contexts: Connect, Be Active, Take Notice, Keep Learning, and Give.

- *Medical and complementary health support*[7] – relating skilfully to your medical team. Appreciating their role in keeping you well and communicating mindfully with them, especially when anxious. Complementary therapies can help in alleviating the side effects of treatment and increasing a sense of personal well-being. Reflecting on the support you get from different sources.

Practice Plans

Having looked at factors that influence daily life, we now develop specific practice plans that address three different contexts.

1 For everyday life.
2 For days when feeling vulnerable.
3 For tough times, when something has occurred that has significant charge, such as a recurrence.

When I first started teaching mindfulness, participants tended to focus on everyday practice plans. I lacked the courage and experience to help them turn towards the reality that difficulty, in whatever form, is an inevitable part of life. As the years went by, I noticed that people often incorporated mindfulness without much awareness of what they were doing. Like Ruth's example earlier, they might bring the breath into everyday life, but it became an automatic habit rather than an aware choice. If a recurrence or some other crisis occurred, their connection with mindfulness was not sufficiently robust or secure to offer them the support they needed.

Now, *turning towards* is an integral part of the program. We always include a plan for tough times. We mention the possibility of recurrence, however much we wish it does not happen. As a result, there seems to be a marked shift in the capacity of people with cancer who attend this mindfulness-based program to stay in touch with their practice, and have it close at hand when they need it.

1   Everyday life practice

Without a clear plan and a strong intention, most of us will not manage to sustain practice. Busyness will take over.

In the light of your current circumstances, can you frame a practice plan that is realistic and interesting?

Regular Practice		
	Which Practices	**When / How often**
CORE		
SHORT		

2   Practice for vulnerable times

There are always going to be days when you feel more vulnerable. Perhaps an annual check-up is coming up. Things you imagined would be straightforward may prove harder than expected. Maybe you have had some sad news. Any number of events or situations can leave us vulnerable to reactivity and stress. Even a poor night's sleep has its impact on mood.

In response to these times, can you frame a daily practice regime that is realistic and kindly? It may just need an extra ingredient, or an intention added to your everyday plans. Remember that ignoring vulnerability holds a risk.

Practice for vulnerable times		
	Which Practices	**When / How often**
CORE		
SHORT		

3 Practice for tough times

This plan is for the periods when you recognize that you are under significant pressure. Perhaps this has developed out of vulnerable times, or maybe something has happened that has tipped you into struggling. When we are in the thick of things, it can be difficult to get enough perspective to remember what to do. This is a plan to pull out when you need it – perhaps to place in your notebook or put on the fridge door or on your computer or phone. It will help you remember what you to do. It is better to act sooner, rather than let things get too severe before putting resources in place.

Tough times practice			
	Which Practices	When / How often	How to remember?
CORE			
SHORT			

How will you remember to bring all these plans into action?

Intention for your practice plans

Choose a way of cultivating an intention for these plans. You might go back to the intentions practice on the website.

Alternatively find your own way – reflecting in your notebook; during a sitting practice; or talking it over with a friend. You now know the value and significance of intention. Connecting to what really matters supports you to commit to regular mindfulness practice.

After treatment for bowel cancer, Colin found his mindfulness practice helped him to manage his anxiety. He liked to practice first thing in the morning. It 'set him up' for the rest of the day, he told me. We reflected on a recent conversation that he had with his friend André, who liked to read a good book for half an hour every evening. 'We were amused by our routines', he said. 'In our younger days, we hated regularity!'

Practice Support

Here are some practical tips for maintaining practice. These are drawn from the experience of a number of people who have established and sustained a regular mindfulness practice.

Supporting core practice
- Find somewhere in the house that becomes your practice place.
- Put a photo or flowers or something significant there that reminds you of your intention.
- Find a time to practice that suits you and stick to it.
- Ask other members of the family to respect your practice time, and not disturb you.
- Leave your phone in another room, choosing not to answer calls or texts while you are practicing.
- Set a clear intention at the start as to how long you will practice, and which practice you will follow.
- Start and end in the same way – remembering your overarching intention at the beginning (what really matters to me) – and appreciating your commitment at the end.
- If there is some person or issue on your heart or in your mind, you can practice for them – dedicating the practice for their benefit.
- Add to this list in your journal, of all the ways that you have found to support your core practice.

Supporting everyday practice
- Link your short practices to particular activities (e.g. standing in mountain while the kettle boils; coming to the breath before getting out of bed; taking a pause before checking emails).
- At the start of the day, form an intention to follow a specific short practice that will support what you need to do that day. (e.g. if you have a hospital appointment, deciding to practice Feet on the Floor and Coming to the Breath, whilst waiting).
- Form an intention at the end of the day to briefly review the day and appreciate all the ways that you have been mindful, however tiny.
- Regularly tuning into your general mind state. Noticing various tendencies (tiredness, busyness, upset, transitions, etc.) that are likely to make you more susceptible to rumination and distress – and 'up' your levels of practice (both short and core) for support as needed. Responding in good time.
- Notice what you practice. These easily become habits that are overlooked. Perhaps choosing a day when you take notice of all the different ways that you 'come back'.

- Create some new everyday practices (e.g. Linda walks mindfully whenever she goes to the shed at the bottom of her garden. Robin always looks up at the sky whenever he leaves the house).
- Notice times when anxious thoughts take you unawares. Find a short practice and form an intention to follow it, so that you have extra support at these times.
- Decide how to manage the deluge of digital information. Choosing how much access you want and sticking to it.

Finding an eight week course

If the time is right, participating on a mindfulness-based eight week program might be a helpful next step. Some of you will have already followed one, perhaps before your diagnosis. As long as you feel well enough, and are confident about the skills and training of the mindfulness teacher offering the course, you may well benefit a lot from taking a further course. People often remark that they get even more out of their second and subsequent courses than they did from the first. This speaks volumes about the ongoing potential of mindfulness-based practice.

If you do not have a mindfulness teacher nearby, there may be other options – such as distance learning, or even an online course. However, many people are climbing onto the mindfulness bandwagon, so it would be wise to check out the background, training, supervision, and approach of teachers offering courses. Just adding 'mindfulness' or 'mindful' in front of a training process does not ensure its integrity or even that it is mindful! In many countries, there are now reputable mindfulness-based centers,[8] which train teachers and deliver courses to the public or to specialist populations.

At this time, there are not many specialist mindfulness-based courses for a cancer population[9]– although your area may be different. It is worth discovering your nearest cancer support centre or cancer charity, if there is one – to see what is offers.

You may need to access an open mindfulness-based program, such as MBSR. This may prove to be a good option, especially if you have finished treatment and are feeling generally well. Practicing alongside others, sharing ideas in a group, and learning to be mindful together can be very helpful – even if other members of the group are facing different challenges to you. People on mindfulness-based programs are encouraged not to share their stories or challenges. The time is needed to focus on learning and practice.

This book can only ever be second best to attending a 'live' group-based mindfulness course. There is such value in learning alongside others and seeing that the way that they suffer in much the same way that we do. Feeling compassion for others, we find it possible to soften to our own struggles.

Finding others to practice with

It helps to practice with others. You may discover a mindfulness sitting group, or a local drop in session. You might consider attending a mindfulness retreat, if you have sufficient confidence and practice experience. There may be apps on your mobile phone or tablet that link you to people practicing. You may join with others further away to form a 'virtual' sitting group, such as via Skype®. There are many creative possibilities.

Renewing your intention

Aspirations may have faded since being diagnosed. Were you in the middle of something, which you had to set aside? It may not be the best option for you now – but it helps to have a direction to head towards, and a focus to dedicate our efforts to.

There is a simple daily practice that embodies this. At the beginning of each day, you mindfully fill a bowl with fresh water. As it is filling, you reflect on your intention for the day. When it is full, you place the bowl of water carefully in the corner of a room. At the end of the day, you take the bowl and mindfully pour away the water. As you do this, you reflect on your day, appreciating any part of what you have enjoyed and achieved – and if you choose to, you can dedicate the benefits of your day to share with others.

Notes

1   Rilke, R.M. (2009)
2   Kabat-Zinn, J. (1995)
3   'The Gift' by Lee, L-Y. (1986)
4   Developed by Trish Bartley and Ursula Bates. The Three Circle Model is included at the back of the book (see Bartley, 2012).
5   Bartley, T. (2012)
6   See www.fivewaystowellbeing.org
7   See https://nccih.nih.gov/health/cancer/camcancer.htm?lang=en#research for up to date research on complementary health therapies and their use with cancer.
8   See Appendix 2 for resources and mindfulness-based centres. However this list is not exhaustive and is constantly being updated.
9   Linda Carlson and her team in Calgary, Canada have been teaching courses and undertaking world class research in MBCR – Mindfulness-Based Cancer Recovery for many years. See Carlson, & Speca, 2011.

And Some More

Standing like a mountain rooted in the ground
Seeing clouds and thoughts drift by
Feeling the wind and the rain
Knowing yesterday has passed
And tomorrow does not exist
There is only now and now and now.

Thoughts may not be reality and that's a fact
And it may not matter if you do or you don't
Just as long as you remember to breathe
To walk mindfully on the earth
And to take the chance to dance with life.

David

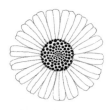

Personal Story

Helen

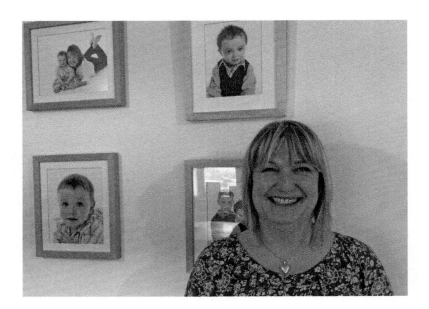

Helen is 46. She lives with her partner and their two boys, 11 and 7. Her partner is a farmer. They live in a lovely part of North Wales. Helen led a team of legal advisers in a magistrate's court for 24 years and really enjoyed it. She gave up work in March 2014 after a recurrence of breast cancer and a poor long-term prognosis. She is currently receiving chemotherapy and doing well.

Mindfulness: A Kindly Approach to Being with Cancer, First Edition. Trish Bartley.
© 2017 John Wiley & Sons, Ltd. Published 2017 by John Wiley & Sons, Ltd.
Companion Website: www.wiley.com/go/bartley/mindfulness

Diagnosis

In July 2008, I found an odd puckering in the nipple region. I didn't expect it to be anything but got it checked out. They found a lobular cancer at the back of the breast. It was quite large at six centimetres.

It was shocking. My youngest was only 18 months old, and I'd not been back at work long. The carpet was really taken out from under me. I stopped work immediately and had to have chemotherapy before surgery.

Treatment

I remember that treatment time in the Day Unit as being quite dark and grim. I can't remember any younger people there. All the other women were quite a lot older. Of course the light, the silver lining, was the nurses there. They kept me going. I remember D, my partner, telling me not to speak to anyone – as the first lady I spoke to had a terminal diagnosis and told me she was keeping herself alive to go to her son's wedding.

I had one sort of chemo for three months and then another sort for another three months. The first three months was ok. I'd be out and about with R at home with me, so I was kept busy. I was fine. I had quite high levels of anxiety but I kept the lid on it and told myself, 'just don't go there'.

I had a lumpectomy in February 2009. They had hoped to preserve the breast, but I didn't really care, to be honest. But Mr. C., the surgeon wasn't able to get sufficient clearance, so I had to go back for a mastectomy. That was really tough. I didn't feel very strong after the first surgery, and the second three months of chemotherapy was awful. I look back on that time and it is like a haze. I felt as if I was in a sort of bubble, distant from the world and everyone – even though friends and family were brilliant.

I then had radiotherapy, which was no problem. I had a different friend or family member taking me in each day. It was quite sociable and I enjoyed that. (*laughing*)

Mindfulness

I started a mindfulness course in May 2009 before going back to work. I remember at the interview in the hospital, you asked me why I wanted to do it. 'I want to force myself to face up to what I've been through, in case it comes back to haunt me', I said. I remember you saying, 'maybe you can be kind to yourself, rather than forcing'. That was the first time I ever considered thinking like that. I need to be kind to myself. I remember that.

People had been telling me, 'you've been brilliant and so brave', but I didn't feel brilliant or brave. I didn't know where I'd been during those last three months of chemo and I needed to know, to find out where I was now. I also didn't think I had the tools to deal with it. I wanted to be better prepared, in case it happened again. Thank God I did!

We had such a good group on the course and there was someone my age. It was lovely. I wrote a poem (*shown at the end of this account*). I still remember it. I wanted to live so much at the time (*crying*) – and I still do – but I'm so grateful for the time I've had. To think that R was only 18 months at the start and I've had all this extra time with him. I'm still here. I'm not going anywhere. I'm not finished yet.

Not a single session went by without somebody saying something that made me think. Each person has his or her own baggage and reason for doing the course. We do the same practices, and learn the same things, but everyone takes from mindfulness what they need.

Second cancer

In 2010, I went for a mammogram and the radiologist saw a shadow. It was another primary. I chose to have a mastectomy. I remember arguing with Mr. C. I told him that I didn't care. Survival is more important than vanity. I didn't need chemo or radiotherapy and started Tamoxifen straight away.

It was a shock to have cancer again, but this one was more straightforward than the first. Tamoxifen brought on the menopause and hot flushes – not very extreme side effects, but still a shock to the system. I was young at 43, and my body was changing. Still – I felt much more connected this time. I felt more able to cope.

I had resources to fall back on. I used all the principles of mindfulness, which had never gone far away. I was still doing the Body Scan now and again. Also I learned to watch myself. Because of my work and the type of person I am – I do a lot of planning ahead – and that is what you mustn't do when you've got cancer. It is so easy to run away with myself and imagine a doom-laden future. That is even more of an issue now. So I would pause and know that there is no factual basis for my thoughts. I could have a look around my body, as it were – and think 'well, I feel ok today.' I've learned that it is best to focus on physical feelings of how you are NOW, to help your mental state.

I went back to work quite quickly in December 2010. I was different this time. I wasn't so ambitious. When I returned to work the first time, I felt different, but quickly fell back into old ways of working too hard, not looking after myself, and taking too much on. The second time, I was definitely different.

I was still doing my best, but I wasn't bringing work home and I was trying to focus on time with the boys, my partner, and my friends.

Recurrence and terminal diagnosis

In February 2012, I had to have a scan and the results came through. That was the worst. I remember asking Dr. B, the oncologist, 'How long do I have?' She said, 'It is very difficult to say – perhaps about two and a half years.' (Isn't it awful for these doctors having to say things like that to people?) I remember thinking, 'that is not enough.'

That diagnosis was really bad. Thankfully, D had insisted on coming with me. We came home and I said to D, 'what do we do now? Where do we go from here?' On the first two times, we had the breast care nurses for support, but this time, we had no one. How do you carry on whilst you have this knowledge that you are going to die? We were in shock and didn't know who we could ring. It was unreal. I took time off work. I wouldn't have been any good to anyone. I was like a zombie for the first few days and then I cried a lot. I couldn't stop crying. I cried mostly on my own, because it was so overwhelming. I kept thinking, 'where do I start?'

Getting help

I had to get some help. I was put in touch with a nurse at another hospital, but on the day she was due, she rang to cancel. She must have thought I was a raving lunatic, because I said to her in desperation on the phone, 'I must see somebody.' I had hung on to see her – so I insisted that I had to see her that day. 'OK, can you get here to the hospital?' she asked. I couldn't drive because I was in such a state, so D drove me and I saw her and just cried and cried. I was absolutely desperate. I was convinced that there was something or somebody out there who could help me. But I didn't know how to go about finding them.

I finally got to J (psycho-oncologist), through this nurse. The minute I walked into her office, I thought 'O, thank God.' She was lovely. I saw her weekly for a while and she helped to steady me and get me out of panic mode.

My boss, who is a great support, said of that time, 'It was like you were on the platform of the station with your case packed, but you didn't know when the train was coming.' I thought I had to do everything I could to prepare myself for death. I don't know why I felt like that. I suppose it is a coping instinct. J told me that I had a safety net around me – you, her and G, from the hospice. I liked that thought and I still feel that now.

Mindfulness In My Life Now

These days, I do the Body Scan still and the Pause, and Coming to the Breath quite a bit. I read a lot. I notice everything a lot more than I used to. Previously I'd be rushing round, planning ahead, thinking about all these things that I have to do. I am still rushing now – but less so – and what I really enjoy is going for a walk with the boys at the weekend. I think 'this is lovely' and really notice the blackberries and the berries in the hedge. It is as if I am imprinting them on my memory – not because I'm being morbid, because I'm quite well at the moment – but because I'm really enjoying the weather, finding things in the hedge, the horse in the field and really noticing.

This is also true with the boys and the funny things they say. R comes out with some marvels. D was saying something to R about when he was grown up. R said when I'm grown up, you're going to be really old!

We haven't told them about the prognosis and I don't know when we will. H knows that I have to take chemotherapy tablets and that they make my feet sore and might make me a bit tired. He knows I've got cancer (I didn't want him to be scared of the 'c' word) but we haven't told them any more than that. Six months is a lifetime to them.

D says I am approaching cancer the same way I would approach a project at work. I've got to know everything there is to know about it. Dying is the current project! I've got all these books. I feel that the more I know, the more control I have – not over the cancer – but over how I react and how I can live with it.

I want to write to the boys. It is going to be quite painful, but quite fun as well. I want to include a section about girls – and tell them not to have sex until they are at least 35!! I'm going to put the letter in a folder, and have it all in their memory boxes. There will be photos as well, and my friend has asked if I want to do a video diary.

My Dad died when I was in my 30s. He just fell down so I don't really have much experience of dying. How wonderful for him. This is a different way and I am doing it my way.

Advice for others in the same boat

I would tell them not to be afraid of living with a terminal prognosis. Just live – and use mindfulness to *really* live your life, instead of just skimming over it. Noticing things, remembering things. Enjoying things as they happen instead of always planning or thinking ahead. Leave the ironing on the ironing table, and go out with the children to play.

Do I live well? Ask yourself the question. Don't be frightened. Have your safety nets in place and just get on with it.

Quite often I think to myself that I must stop talking to people about cancer. It is very easy to become self-centered. There are other things in the world apart from me and cancer!

I Just Want to Live … …

'I just want to live…..', I said
when told I had cancer.
'I'll do anything …'
I poisoned my body with chemo.
I disfigured it with two operations.
I burnt my body with radiotherapy
All because
I just wanted to live.

'I just want to live …'
'Yes, yes,' she said, 'but why not try a different way?
Why not try living with
Awareness
Love
Kindness
Peace?'

Because now I don't just want to live,
I want to live with meaning and with feeling.
So thank you for starting this journey with me,
And whatever happens in future,
May we all go in peace.
Because at the end of the day,
We all want to live.

Helen

Chapter 6
Connecting To Our Common Humanity

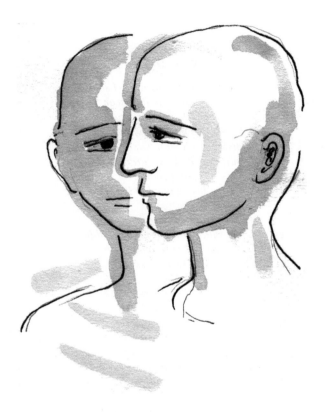

A person is not basically an independent solitary entity. A person is human precisely in being enveloped in the community of other human beings, in being caught up in the bundle of life ... not independence, but interdependence.[1]

Desmond Tutu

Mindfulness: A Kindly Approach to Being with Cancer, First Edition. Trish Bartley.
© 2017 John Wiley & Sons, Ltd. Published 2017 by John Wiley & Sons, Ltd.
Companion Website: www.wiley.com/go/bartley/mindfulness

We have been cultivating a sense of connection with those like us—reading alongside, sitting alongside, receiving treatment alongside, and sometimes suffering alongside. Others like us wait for results, appointments, side effects to pass, anxiety to abate – just as we have. Around the world, many millions like us are going through similar times, albeit in different hospitals and health systems.

Putting ourselves in the shoes of those who suffer, our compassion naturally flows.

Learning To Live With Uncertainty

Planned routines, such as the practice plans you created from the previous chapter, are helpful when they are backed by wise intentions. However, sticking rigidly to a plan while expecting a particular result only perpetuates the myth that we are in control. It is what we do, but it is the cause of many of our struggles.

Accepting that life is profoundly uncertain is not about giving up – quite the reverse. It is to find the space inside a moment of 'not-knowing' that holds promise of blessed relief. We can put down the burden of trying so hard. We can rest in a place that acknowledges both the wish to control and our inability to do so – and find moments of ease that this is how it is. It is ultimately freeing.

Like the cadence of falling leaves in autumn, we untangle ourselves from the 'knots of our own making'.

Reflecting on change

That brooding anxiety ... ... its quivering unease is like the lazy collision of two rings of ripples on water: one reverberation from the shock of birth, the other an intimation of the shock of death.[2]

Mindfulness practice teaches us to be aware of the detail of moment by moment change, in the body and around us. We bring attention to the subtle and not so subtle shifts in nature – noticing the transition of the seasons; the changing weather; the evolving colours on the hills and in the garden. Yet, we do not quite take on board that the nature of everything is essentially transient and temporary. We fix things with labels and concepts that in reality are constantly in process.

This holds true for us too. We feel that this 'me' has an enduring identity. People often say that they want to get the 'old me' back after being ill – but I suspect that few feel they do. Our lives are profoundly altered when we become 'patients' and go through treatment. Life threatening illness is bound to change us – but every experience does too. Having treatment for cancer simply brings this into a sharper focus.

> *It is not that the self does not exist, but that it is as cobbled together and transient as everything else.*[3]

Instead of resisting the process of change, and trying to claw a way back to where we used to be, can we allow things to be, as they are now? Can we allow ourselves to be, as we are now? There may be nothing to be done and trying hard to make it otherwise may prove exhausting. Letting go of the fight, we can play with the possibility of resting in the preciousness of being alive in this moment, now.

> *We tend to forget that life can only be defined in the present tense.*[4]

Facing Mortality, Finding Life

> *Life-threatening illness calls us to a place – metaphorical desert or mountain peak – where, as we sit, the hard wind of reality strips away all the trappings of life … … (and) we are left naked.*[5]

Some of you, reading this book, may know that you are moving closer to dying. All of us are in that position, but those with terminal illness are forced into an awareness of mortality that is sharper and closer. The rest of us manage to skirt around this, most of the time.

Wherever you are with this, reflecting on the transience of life and the inevitability of death, can support the business of living – strange as that may sound. Perhaps we can turn the experience of illness, past or present, into an opportunity to bring meaning and impetus into how we live and how relate to each other, now.

A colleague went on a course about dying. A bit to her surprise, the focus was personal not professional. They were asked to imagine they could choose the manner of their death. Most people wanted to die in their beds or after a short illness. They argued that this would limit their suffering, and reduce the likelihood of being a burden on their families. My colleague 'chose' to die of a progressive illness. She reasoned that this would give her a chance to say goodbye to loved ones, put her affairs in order, and resolve any outstanding difficulties. She was surprised to find that some of the others were won over to her 'corner'.

What do you make of this story?

At the beginning of this book, you were invited to ask:

> *What really matters to me?*

We return to this question now. If you knew that you only had a few weeks or so to live, what would matter to you?

> *You never know how much you really believe anything until its truth or false-hood becomes a matter of life and death to you."*[6]

Contemplating the end-of-life can be an opportunity to reassess priorities, and stop delaying our lives. It may be a tragedy to live life on automatic pilot and not realize what we have been doing until too late.

Birth plans do not guarantee a good delivery, but they are still worth doing. The same is true of envisaging how you would like to die, which after all can include a broad range of experience from deep suffering to wellness and peace.

> *Death may live in the living and healing rise in the dying.*[7]

Perhaps, as in life, much depends on how we relate to the experience – and in the care we are offered. Some describe dying as a developmental process, where the world keeps shifting with fresh challenges to negotiate. Insecurity is a constant. Relationships change. There are many obvious physical challenges. None of this sounds appealing and managing it can clearly involve struggle. But like much else – indeed like cancer itself – perhaps dying can be an opportunity to open to vulnerability and move back into being held and cared for, if we are fortunate. Could it also be a time for giving and receiving kindness?

All that we have learnt about living mindfully can be put to use in the process of dying.

Beth lay very ill in the hospice. Her breath was laboured and she was evidently moving closer to death. Peggy came to sit beside her. She had taught Beth mindfulness and had supported her during the latter stages of her illness. She reached out to hold her hand. 'He's telling me to breathe', Beth whispered to her, 'I can hear his voice saying "Just breathe".' It took Peggy some moments to realize that Beth was not hallucinating, or having some religious experience – but referring to Jon Kabat-Zinn's voice on the mindfulness recordings they used.

'Let's breathe together', Peggy suggested.

Part of the art of dying, as in living, seems to involve talking about the things we usually avoid. There may be deep pain in such a final loss, but it may also be an opportunity to heal rifts within the family and to acknowledge and appreciate significant connections, even as the withdrawing and parting is occurring.

Dorothy was a South African hospice nurse. They were always short of beds in the hospice for so many were dying of Aids. She went to visit a very sick woman in one of the townships on the outskirts of town. She found her lying unwashed in an unsanitary condition, close to death, with no running water close by. Dorothy had been taught that dignity in death was paramount. To her, this poor woman was dying in a terribly undignified way. Yet she was deeply moved by the presence of the woman's neighbours who were gathered around the simple bed singing her out as she died. 'It was such a paradox', Dorothy told me, her voice breaking with emotion. 'There was so little dignity, and yet so much love.'

Pausing here before we move on – to feel the feet on the floor, to breathe, to feel what you are feeling … … to take your time.

Some areas you might want to reflect on

I have outlined some tasks and issues that you might want to reflect on. Developing ideas about what you might want in your last days is a way of turning towards the impermanence of life. Those who do this, tell us that it helps them live the life they want now.

When we turn mindfully to the idea that we are going to die, we stop delaying our lives.[8]

Choose a time when this feels appropriate. There is no need to rush into it.

Practical and legal matters
- drawing up/updating your will
- reflect on your medical care wishes (advanced medical directives involve different regulations in different countries)
- letting your next of kin know the location of your legal documents (e.g., house deeds, financial papers, will, wishes book, passwords, etc.)
- share instructions for burial or cremation, funeral, etc.

Loved ones – memory boxes? Personal gifts or mementos? Letters?
Unfinished business – this may cover a range of issues, from disagreements with people, to legal matters, and even to de-cluttering the house.

This second group relate to what might nourish and support your last days.

Place – hospice, home or hospital?
Music – pieces, composers, CDs, genres (what would be your '8 desert island discs'?)
Readings – poetry, stories, religious readings
Smells – fragrances or none
People – family members, friends, pets
Sights – special photos or pictures
Practices – guided practices

What might help us to die peacefully? Much of it is out of our hands. We cannot know how things will be. We may die in our sleep or have time to make farewells. How we relate to our dying will have an influence on how our family members relate to each other after we have gone. What might support you to be generous and honest in your living, as in your dying?

How can we make the most of the time we have left?

No Lovely Words

When we went outside into the sun,
to find something that spoke
of what we were taking away,
I found myself choosing a lily
that on close inspection was dead, clearly dead.

Why would I do such a thing?

In a moment, I thought to cheat.
Drop this one and choose the next,
a real beauty with its white full petals,
cream tinged, blue and yellow throated.

I could tell of the riches I felt,
of the joy of knowing them.
It would be superb, my little speech!

And even as the words formed
in their cadences and crescendos,
I knew I would not.

No lovely words then,
as I walked back along the path,
heavy hearted into that lovely dark room.

But somewhere,
in the walking and the coming back of it,
I looked inside my wizened lily,
and saw something more lovely
than the most perfect of them all.

I was not finished here.
I would be back.
For in every dead thing
are there not the seeds of the next?

North Wales, August 2013

Living Mindfully

Three key themes run through this book.

- The first is the *embodiment of mindfulness* brought into everyday life to ease our struggles and grow contentment and calm.
- The second is the *cultivation of kindness* that opens the heart and softens to the pain that lies within.
- The third is the *remembering* in heart, body and mind that *we are not alone.*

Others suffer, just like me.
Others feel alone, just like me.
Others have to manage the business of living and dying, just like me.
Others can rest in the beauty of the world and be free, just like me.

In Africa, this connection with 'others like me' is known as Ubuntu. 'I am who I am, because of you, and who you are'. It speaks of our interconnectedness. In rural Africa, village people relate to their extended family as mothers and fathers, sisters and brothers. This is not just a social convention. It has important practical significance. When your brother or sister is struggling with illness, poverty, or hunger, if you can, you help out. When I lived in South Africa, I heard of people giving precious scarce food to a neighbour. Others like me.

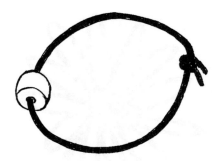

The thread that we use in the 'cancer' practices was first created for people affected by HIV and Aids in South Africa. They are now worn and shared in mindfulness sessions, in many different contexts and countries. I wanted a thread to be tucked into each of these books, but it was not possible. I always wear a thread myself and many hundreds and possibly thousands of people do too. If you wear a thread, you can connect with everyone else who is also wearing one – and even if you do not, you can still connect with everyone practicing mindfulness like you. You can wish them well in your heart, knowing that they wish *you* well.

Maybe we can play with the possibility that what we do in our practice of mindfulness affects far more than we imagine. The ripples that spread out may continue spreading a long way, for a long time – into families and friends, medical teams and colleagues – and out further to connect with all those others like us, well and ill, living and dying, young and old, black and white. Wishing them well.

Notes

1   See http://uwi-usa.blogspot.be/2012/01/ubuntu-brief-meaning-of-african-word.html
2   Batchelor, S. (2004)
3   Olendzki, A. (2010)
4   Interview with Melvyn Bragg. Channel 4 Television, UK. (March 1994, shortly before his death) see Potter, D. (1994).
5   Byock, I. (2008) Foreword in Joan Halifax's *Being with Dying*.
6   Lewis, C.S. (1961)
7   Torrie, M. (1984)
8   Levine, S. (1992) *An interview with Stephen Levine*, Reproduced in the week of his death 17 January 2016.

The Raku Bowl

Like a raku bowl
that goes into the dark
without mould or cast,
a true warrior lives
and dies with uncertainty,
knows how to reconcile
two halves of the whole,
knows that to be vulnerable
is like the fragile beauty
of a vessel holding life
on the edge of breaking.

So from a lost crow's nest,
the iridescence
of a bird of paradise
is found.

Jill Teague
Maentwrog, North Wales

Some Parting Words

I have often brought you to mind as I have been writing this book. I am curious about you. Where do you come from? How have you managed the particulars of your journey? What has it offered you?

I wonder too how these chapters have landed with you. I do not need to know – but your presence has been around during these many months of writing. You have changed gender and race, age and stage of cancer. You have morphed into all the people I have ever taught. They line up, arriving at different times, reminding me of what was significant to them, repeating snatches of our conversations, of their experience, of their courage, practicing together with them. I hope they have offered you some sense of connection, as well.

As I have neared the end of this, I have been struck at how similar we are. We are all challenged by the stories of the mind – all faced by changing, aging bodies and uncertain futures. This sounds pretty gloomy, until I recollect that apart from the specifics of cancer, this is true for all humans. We, none of us, know when we will die. We all have losses and worries that wake us in the night (and if you are not one of these, you probably have other trials). Yet, we all have the potential to live life well – to be fulfilled, to find meaning, to care deeply, whatever the current state of our health.

Out of the darkness of illness and struggle can come an opportunity to deepen and develop practice, to better understand the ways of suffering, and to appreciate all the more what matters most.

Mindfulness: A Kindly Approach to Being with Cancer, First Edition. Trish Bartley.
© 2017 John Wiley & Sons, Ltd. Published 2017 by John Wiley & Sons, Ltd.
Companion Website: www.wiley.com/go/bartley/mindfulness

I have been concerned to avoid falling into the trap of presenting practice as straightforward or easy. There are days when I need to dig deep to get onto my practice 'cushion' – but I cannot remember one time that I have later regretted, or considered there was something better I could have done. Sometimes, it has been difficult to offer you an authentic balance between optimism and realism – that razors edge of describing possibilities that are neither too upbeat, nor too grim. Whenever I have misjudged this, as I am bound to have done at times, I apologize. I hope it has not hindered your learning.

Does my practice and commitment to mindfulness mean that I no longer feel anxious and alone at times? No – fear and anxiety still visit me, especially when my mind is busy with some issue or other. The difference is that I now have resources to draw on. I tend to have a softer way of relating to myself and my world. I enjoy my life and the people within it a lot more. I am not quite so definite!

I notice and enjoy more of 'the small moments', which as Jon Kabat-Zinn says:

The small moments are not so small – they're life[1]!

And what of you? If you were to write a letter to all those who have been travelling with you, in the clinics, the treatment rooms, hospital beds, radiotherapy suites and in all the countless waiting areas – what would you tell them? What have you encountered in the 'wilderness' of your mind that might help them with theirs? If you were to describe the nuggets of your discovered truths – what shape might they be? What would you say now about love? What would you sing to the trees?

North Wales, July 2016

[1] Jon Kabat-Zinn (1993) Interview with Bill Moyers.

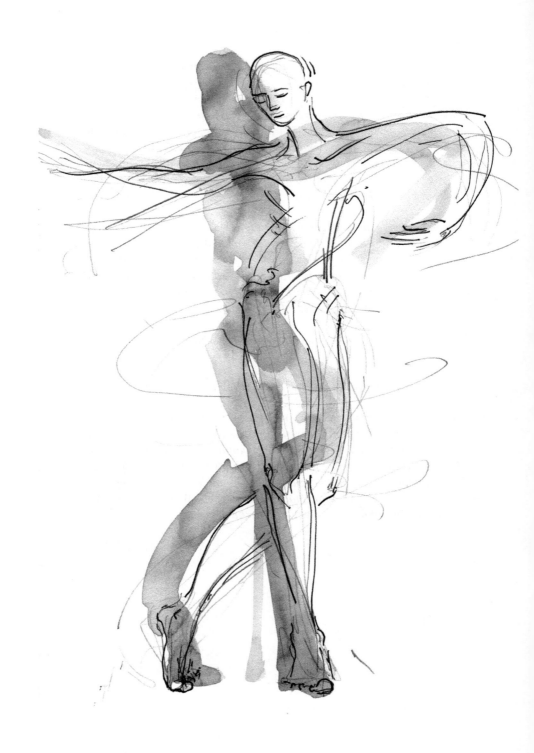

Appendix 1

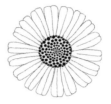

Cancer And Mindfulness-Based Approaches

Brief Research Headlines

Mindfulness-based cancer recovery (MBCR)

Linda E. Carlson has been undertaking research into Mindfulness for people with cancer since 2000. If you would like to read about the evidence for this approach, Linda's website is the place to go. She and her team are based at the University of Calgary, Alberta, Canada and within the Tom Baker Integrative Oncology Centre. They have undertaken a vast range of research and have established an evidence base for the benefit of mindfulness for people with cancer. Their work in this field is extraordinarily significant.

Linda Carlson and her team researched Mindfulness-Based Cancer Recovery (MBCR) and compared it to Supportive Expressive Therapy (SET) (Carlson, et al., 2013) and found MBCR to be superior for improving a range of psychological outcomes for distressed survivors of breast cancer.

This website lists all their research publications: https://lindacarlson.ca

Mindfulness-based stress reduction (MBSR)

Caroline Hoffman undertook a randomised research trial (RCT) in the UK (Hoffman et al., 2012) with 214 breast cancer patients and found their mood, quality of life and well-being improved significantly. This research found new

Mindfulness: A Kindly Approach to Being with Cancer, First Edition. Trish Bartley.
© 2017 John Wiley & Sons, Ltd. Published 2017 by John Wiley & Sons, Ltd.
Companion Website: www.wiley.com/go/bartley/mindfulness

evidence that MBSR can help alleviate long-term emotional and physical adverse effects of treatment.

Mindfulness-based cognitive therapy (MBCT)

Elizabeth Foley undertook a randomised research trial (RCT) in Australia (Foley et al., 2010) investigating MBCT for 115 people with a range of different sites and stages of cancer. She found that MBCT offered improvement in levels of depression, anxiety and distress. These results were sustained at a three-month follow up.

Christina Shennan reviewed all the available evidence for mindfulness-based interventions in cancer care. Her article (Shennan, Payne & Fenlon, 2011) is available online and although there are more up to date reviews available, this one is well thought of, and a good place to start.

There are a growing number of research trials and studies into mindfulness-based interventions in cancer care. This is only a snapshot of what is currently out there as I write. Happily, the evidence for the effectiveness of mindfulness-based interventions for cancer care is established and growing.

Appendix 2

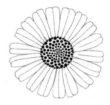

Resources

This list is based on the organizations I work with or know something about.

Look at the Good Practice Guidelines for internationally accepted good practice standards in mindfulness-based teaching.
Available at http://www.mindfulnessteachersuk.org.uk

United Kingdom

Centre for Mindfulness, Research and Practice (CMRP)
www.bangor.ac.uk/mindfulness

Oxford Mindfulness Centre (OMC)
www.oxfordmindfulness.org

Exeter Mindfulness Network
www.cedar.exeter.ac.uk/mindfulness

Breathworks – *mindfulness courses in groups and online, for people living with pain, stress and illness. Based in the UK with teachers in many parts of the world.*
www.breathworks-mindfulness.org.uk

Mindfulness: A Kindly Approach to Being with Cancer, First Edition. Trish Bartley.
© 2017 John Wiley & Sons, Ltd. Published 2017 by John Wiley & Sons, Ltd.
Companion Website: www.wiley.com/go/bartley/mindfulness

Mindfulness Network CIC – *MBSR and MBCT courses and retreats delivered by teachers who have met the UK Good Practice Guidelines.*
www.mindfulness-network.org

The Mindfulness Initiative – *works with UK parliament, media and policy makers. Informative website re mindfulness in the UK and further afield.*
www.themindfulnessinitiative.org.uk

UK Network for Mindfulness-Based Teacher Training Organisations – list *of UK mindfulness-based teachers who have met Good Practice Guidelines (GPG).*
www.mindfulnessteachersuk.org.uk

Australasia

Mindfulness Training Institute, Australasia
www.mtia.org.au

South Africa

The Institute for Mindfulness South Africa
www.mindfulness.org.za

The Netherlands

Mindfulness-Based Trainers in the Netherlands (VMBM)
http://www.vmbn.nl/

See True Training
www.mindfulness-opleiding.nl

United States

Centre for Mindfulness in Medicine, Health Care and Society (CFM)
www.umassmed.edu/cfm

The UC San Diego Center for Mindfulness (UCSD)
www.ucsdcfm.wordpress.com

Web Links

Mindfulness-Based Cancer Recovery – at Tom Baker Cancer Centre, Alberta.
www.tbbcintegrative.com
www.lindacarlson.ca

Mindfulness-Based Cognitive Therapy (North America)
www.mbct.com

Other useful web links

Akincano Marc Weber – a number of his talks are available at: www.dharmaseed.org

Christina Feldman – a number of her talks are available at: www.dharmaseed.org

Mindfulness in Schools Project and.b. Information on this is available at https://mindfulnessinschools.org/

Thought on a thread. Available at: www.thoughtonathread.co.uk

Trigonos, North Wales – a lovely centre where many mindfulness-based retreats take place. See: www.trigonos.org

www.fivewaystowellbeing.org – an evidence based project that highlights five ways to wellbeing

www.mariahayes.info – Maria has drawn the two full-page illustrations at the front and the back of the book – Closing and Opening – and also the last chapter illustration.

Appendix 3

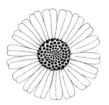

The Three Circle Model of Mindfulness-Based Cognitive Therapy for Cancer (MBCT-Ca)

This is a 'map' of MBCT for Cancer and the approach of this book. It is a diagram that seeks to represent the key features of the MBCT-Ca approach.

The first circle outlines the psychological impact of cancer – that includes **Trauma**; **Rumination**; **Avoidance** and **Distress**. The second circle illustrates the intervention of mindfulness, with the four movements that we use to structure the learning in this book – **Intention**; **Coming Back**; **Turning Towards** and **Kindness**. The final circle proposes four qualities – **Embodying** the ground of experience; **Appreciating** the richness of experience; **Confident to be with** experience; and **Connecting** to our common humanity

Ursula Bates and Trish Bartley developed this formulation. If you would like to read more about it – see *Mindfulness-Based Cognitive Therapy for Cancer* (Bartley, 2012).

The two illustrations at the front and back of this book, created beautifully by Maria Hayes, are representations of 'closing' and 'opening' as pointed to by the arrows in the Three Circle Model overleaf

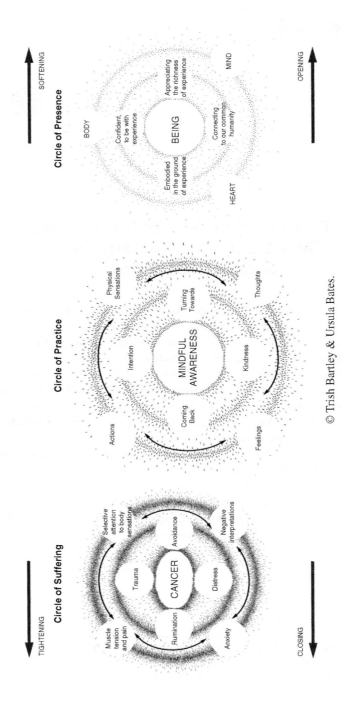

Circle of Suffering

TIGHTENING

CLOSING

Selective attention to body sensations

Muscle tension and pain

Trauma

Avoidance

CANCER

Rumination

Distress

Negative interpretations

Anxiety

Circle of Practice

Physical Sensations

Turning Towards

Thoughts

Intention

MINDFUL AWARENESS

Kindness

Actions

Coming Back

Feelings

Circle of Presence

SOFTENING

OPENING

BODY

MIND

Appreciating the richness of experience

Confident, to be with experience

BEING

Connecting to our common humanity

Embodied in the ground of experience

HEART

© Trish Bartley & Ursula Bates.

Appendix 4

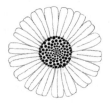

Lee Watson, talented chef and author, *beachhousekitchen.com* has kindly created three soups for us. Maybe you can choose to cook them mindfully, being aware of the colours, sounds, smells and tastes as you prepare and eat them.

SQUASH AND SESAME SOUP

You can keep the squash seeds and roast them in an oven.

The Bits – Two large bowlfuls

750 g squash/1 medium squash (peeled, de-seeded and cut into small, 2 cm chunks)
1 large onion (sliced)
4–6 large cloves garlic (peeled and crushed) (optional)
2 teaspoons cumin seeds
1 teaspoon turmeric
750 mL hot water
½ teaspoon salt
2–3 tablespoon tahini
2 tablespoons rapeseed oil (or other oil)

Garnish

2 tablespoons toasted sesame seeds

Mindfulness: A Kindly Approach to Being with Cancer, First Edition. Trish Bartley.
© 2017 John Wiley & Sons, Ltd. Published 2017 by John Wiley & Sons, Ltd.
Companion Website: www.wiley.com/go/bartley/mindfulness

Add the oil to a large saucepan on a medium high heat. Warm the oil for a minute, add the cumin seeds and allow them to cook for 30 seconds. Add the onions, then the salt and stir. Fry for five minutes, add the garlic, stir and cook for two minutes more.

Now add the squash and turmeric, stir well and pour over the water or stock. Bring to a boil and lower the heat to a gentle simmer. Pop a lid on a leave to cook for 20 minutes.

Stir in the tahini (to taste) and blend with a stick blender until smooth. Pop the lid back on and allow to simmer gently for a couple of minutes more.

Serve topped with a scattering of toasted sesame seeds.

CREAMY ROASTED TOMATO, RED PEPPER AND BASIL

The Bits – Two bowlfuls

12 medium tomatoes (cut in half)
2 red peppers (cut in half and deseeded)
1 large onion (sliced)
1 large bulb garlic (top trimmed off to just expose cloves) (optional)
2 handfuls fresh basil leaves
1 tin coconut milk
1–2 tablespoons balsamic vinegar
2 teaspoons olive oil
Salt and pepper

Garnish

More basil leaves
Chilli flakes (optional)

Preheat oven to 180 °C.

Lightly oil a large baking tray and add tomatoes, pepper and garlic. Place in the oven and roast for 35 minutes. The garlic should be soft.

In a saucepan, add a splash of olive oil and on a medium heat, fry your onions until softened.

Pop the garlic cloves out of their skins and add the tomatoes, peppers and garlic to the saucepan along with the coconut milk. Simmer for 10 minutes on a low heat. Add the balsamic vinegar and basil leaves.

Now blend the soup using a stick blender or pour into a food processor and blitz until smooth. Season with salt and pepper, adding a touch more balsamic if you like.

Serve in warm bowls, garnishing with extra basil leaves, freshly ground pepper and some chilli flakes (if you like a little chilli kick!).

HEALTHY GREENS, GINGER AND MISO BROTH

The Bits – for 6 good bowlfuls

2 medium-sized leeks (finely sliced – using the green part)
1 ½ inch fresh ginger (finely diced)
½ medium savoy cabbage or 4 large handfuls kale
150 g dark green/puy lentils (rinsed)
600 mL warm vegetable stock/water
1 teaspoon dried rosemary
1 teaspoon sunflower oil
1 teas toasted sesame oil (optional)
1 small head broccoli (cut into small florets – using the stem)
6 big handfuls spinach leaves
4–6 tablespoons brown miso (to taste)
sea salt (if needed)

Do It

In a large heavy bottomed saucepan on medium heat, drizzle in the oils and when warm add the leeks and ginger. Fry gently for a few minutes, until soft. Add the cabbage, lentils, stock/water and rosemary to the pan. Bring to a boil and lower heat to a steady simmer, pop a lid on and cook for 25–30 minutes, until the lentils are soft.

Add the broccoli and pop the lid back on, cook for a further 5 minutes on a low simmer. Stir in the spinach leaves and the miso to taste, adding a little hot water to thin out as needed.

Pop the lid back on the saucepan, take off the heat and leave the soup to stand for a couple of minutes. Miso is really like salt with benefits. It will deepen the flavor and add nutrition.

Bibliography

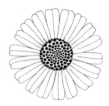

Bartley, T. (2003) *Holding up the sky: Love power and learning in the development of a community*. London: Community Links.

Bartley, T. (2012) *Mindfulness-based cognitive therapy for cancer: Gently turning towards*. Oxford: Wiley-Blackwell.

Batchelor, S. (1990) *The faith to doubt*. Berkeley, CA: Counterpoint.

Batchelor, S. (2001) *Meditation for Life* London: Francis Lincoln.

Batchelor, S. (2004) *Living with the Devil: A meditation on good and evil*. USA: Riverhead Books.

Bates, T. (2005) The expression of compassion in group cognitive therapy. In P. Gilbert (Ed), *Compassion* (p. 379). Hove and New York: Routledge.

Bauer-Wu, S. (2011) *Leaves falling gently: Living fully with serious and life limiting illness through mindfulness, compassion and connectedness*. Oakland, CA: New Harbinger.

Beck, A.T., Rush, A.J., Shaw, B.F., Emery, G. (1979) *Cognitive therapy for depression*. New York: Guilford.

Buber, M. (1958) *I and thou*. 2nd edition. (R. Gregory Smith, Trans.). Edinburgh: T. & T. Clark.

Burch, V. (2008) *Living well with pain and illness: The mindful way to free yourself from suffering*. London: Piatkus.

Burch, V., & Penlan, D. (2013). *Mindfulness for health*. London: Piatkus.

Byock, I. (2008) Foreword in Joan Halifax's *Being with dying*. Shambhala Publications.

Calhoun, L.G., & Tedeschi, R.G. (Eds) (2006, 2014). *Handbook of post traumatic growth: research and practice*. New York and London: Psychology Press.

Carlson, L.E., & Speca, M. (2011) *Mindfulness-based cancer recovery*. Oakland, CA: New Harbinger.

Carlson, L.E., Labelle, L.E., Garlend, S.N., et al. (2009) Mindfulness-based interventions in oncology. In F. Didonna, (Ed.) *Clinical handbook of mindfulness*. New York: Springer (pp. 383–404).

Chödrön, P. (1991) *The wisdom of no escape and the path of loving kindness*. Boston & London: Shambhala Publications.

Chödrön, P. (1997). *When things fall apart: Heart advice for difficult times*. Boston & London: Shambhala Publications.

Clark, A. (2014, September 06) Ali Smith: 'There are two ways to read this novel, but you're stuck with it – you'll end up reading one of them' How to Be Both. [Review of the book *How to Be Both* by A. Smith]. The Guardian. Retrieved from http://www.theguardian.com/books/2014/sep/06/ali-smith-interview-how-to-be-both

Feldman, C. (2005) *Compassion: Listening to the cries of the world*. Berkeley, CA: Rodmell Press.

Foley, E., Baillie, A., Huxter, M., et al. (2010) Mindfulness-based cognitive therapy for individuals whose lives have been affected by Cancer: A randomised controlled trial. *Journal of Consulting and Clinical Psychology*. 78(1), 72–79.

Frankl, V.E. (1959/1984) *Man's search for meaning: An introduction to logotherapy*. New York: Simon & Schuster/Touchstone.

Fredrickson, B. L. & Branigan, C (2005). Positive emotions broaden the scope of attention and thought-action repertoires. *Cognition & Emotion* 19(3), 313–332.

Gawande, A. (2014) *Being mortal: Illness, medicine, and what matters in the end*. London: Wellcome Collection.

Gilbert, P. (2009) *The compassionate mind*. London: Constable.

Goldberg, N. (1986) *Writing down the bones: Freeing the writer within*. Boston: Shambhala Publications.

Goldstein, J. (2002) *ONE Dharma: The emerging western Buddhism*. San Francisco: HarperCollins.

Goldstein, J. (2013) *Mindfulness: A practical guide to awakening*. Boulder, CO: Sounds True.

Gross, K. (2015) *Late fragments: Everything I want to tell you (about this magnificent life)*. London: William Collins.

Hahn, T.N. (2005) *Being peace*. Berkeley, California. Parallax Press.

Halifax, J. (2008) *Being with dying: Cultivating compassion and fearlessness in the presence of death*. Boston: Shambhala Publications.

Hanson, R., & Mendius, R. (2009) *Buddha's brain*. Oakland, CA: New Harbinger.

Hoffman, C.J., Ersser, S.J., Hopkinson, J.B., et al. (2012). Effectiveness of mindfulness based stress reduction in mood, breast- and endocrine-related quality of life, and well-being in stage 0 to III breast cancer: a randomized, controlled trial. *Journal of Clinical Oncology* 30, 1335–1342.

James, C. (2015) *Sentenced to life. Poems 2011–2014*. London: Picador.

Kabat-Zinn, J. (1990, 2013) *Full catastrophe living: Using the wisdom if your body and mind to face stress, pain and illness*. New York: Delta.

Kabat-Zinn, J. (1994). *Wherever you go, there you are: Mindfulness meditation in everyday life*. New York: Hyperion.

Kabat-Zinn, J. (1995) Meditation. In B. Moyers (Ed.) (pp. 115–144). *Healing and the Mind*. New York: Broadway Books.

Kabat-Zinn, M., & Kabat-Zinn, J. (1997, 2014) *Everyday blessings: Mindfulness for parents*. London: Piatkus.

Kalanithi, P. (2016) *When Breath Becomes Air*. London: Random House.

Killingsworth, A.M., & Gilbert, D.T. (2010) A wandering mind is an unhappy mind. *Science*, 330, 932. doi:10.1126

Kornfield, J. (1993) *A Path with heart: Guide through the perils and promises of spiritual life*. New York: Bantam Books.

Lee, L-Y. (1986) *Rose*. New York: BOA Editions.

Levine, S (1992) *No second-guessing: An interview with Stephen Levine*. Tricycle magazine 2, 48–50.

Levine, S. (1987) *Healing into life and death*. Bath: Gateway Books.

Lewis, C.S. (1961) *A grief observed*. London: Faber & Faber.

Macmillan Cancer Support. (2007) *Worried sick – the emotional impact of cancer*. Retrieved from http://www.macmillan.org.uk/documents/getinvolved/campaigns/campaigns/impact_of_cancer_english

Mayne, M. (1995) *This sunrise of wonder: Letters for the journey*. London: Fount.

Michaels, A. (1997) *Fugitive pieces*. London: Bloomsbury.

Moorey, S., & Greer, S. (2002, 2012) *Oxford guide to CBT for people with cancer..* Oxford: Oxford University Press.

Neff, K. (2011) *Self compassion*. London: Hodder & Stoughton.

Nyanasobhano, B. (1998) *Landscapes of wonder*. Somerville, MA: Wisdom.

Olendzki, A. (2010) *Unlimiting Mind*. Somerville, MA: Wisdom.

Owen, R. (2011) *Facing the storm: Using CBT, mindfulness and acceptance to build resilience when your world's falling apart*. Hove, East Sussex: Routledge.

Potter, D. (1994) (Much loved British playwright.) *Without walls*. Interview with Melvyn Bragg. Channel 4 Television, UK.

Remen, R.N. (1996) *Kitchen table wisdom*. New York: Riverhead Books.

Remen, R.N. (2000) *My grandfather's blessings: Stories of strength, refuge and belonging*. New York: Riverhead Books.

Rilke, R.M. (1934) *Letters to a young poet*. (M.D. Herter Norton, Trans.). New York: W.W. Norton.

Rilke, R.M. (1996) *Rilke's book of hours: Love poems to God*. (A. Barrows & J. Macy, Trans.). New York: Riverhead.

Rilke, R.M. (2009) *Early Journals*. (J. Macy and A. Barrows, Trans.). New York: Harper Collins.

Rogers, C.R. (1974) *On becoming a person*. London: Constable.

Rosenbaum, E. (2005) *Here for now: Living well with cancer through mindfulness*. Hardwick, MA: Satya House.

Rosenberg, L., & Guy, D. (1998) *Breath by breath: The liberating practice of insight meditation*. Boston: Shambhala.

Rumi, J.B. (1999) *The essential Rumi* (C. Barks, J. Moyne, A.J. Arberry, & R. Nicholson, Trans.). London and New York: Penguin Books.

Searle, R. (2010) *Les très riches heures de Mrs. Mole*. London: HarperCollins.

Segal, Z.V., Williams, J.M.G., & Teasdale, J.D. (2013) *Mindfulness-based cognitive therapy for depression: A new approach to preventing relapse*. 2nd Edition. New York: The Guilford Press.

Shapiro, S.L., & Carlson, L.E. (2009) *The art and science of mindfulness: Integrating mindfulness into psychology and the helping professions.* Washington: American Psychological Association.

Shennan, C., Payne, S., & Fenlon, D. (2010) What is the evidence for the use of mindfulness-based interventions in cancer care? A review. *Psycho-Oncology* 20(7), 681–697. Retrieved from: http://transformationalchange.pbworks.com/w/file/fetch/55259548/mindful%20in%20cancer.pdf

Suzuki, S. (1973) *Zen mind, beginner's mind.* New York and Tokyo: Weatherhill.

Tarrant, J. (1998) *The light inside the dark: Zen, soul, and the spiritual life.* New York: HarperCollins.

Teasdale, J., Williams, M., & Segal, Z. (2014) *The mindful way workbook: An 8-week program to free yourself from depression and emotional distress.* New York: Guilford.

Teasdale, J.D., & Chaskalson, M. (2011) How does mindfulness transform suffering? 1 & 2. *Contemporary Buddhism.* 12(1), 89–124.

Thomas, R.S. (1993) *Collected poems 1945–1990.* London: Orion Book.

Torrie, M. (1984) *All in the end is harvest.* London: DLT/Cruse.

Tutu, D. (2000) *No future without forgiveness: A personal overview of South Africa's truth and reconciliation commission.* London: Rider.

Whitaker, A. (1984) *All in the end is harvest: An anthology for those who grieve.* London: Darton, Longman & Todd.

Wilber, K. (1991) *Grace and grit.* Boston: Shambhala Publications.

Williams, M., & Penman, D. (2011) *Mindfulness: A practical guide to finding peace in a frantic world.* London: Piatkus.

Index

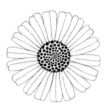

Mindfulness: A Kindly Approach to Being with Cancer, First Edition. Trish Bartley.
© 2017 John Wiley & Sons, Ltd. Published 2017 by John Wiley & Sons, Ltd.
Companion Website: www.wiley.com/go/bartley/mindfulness

About the Author

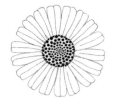

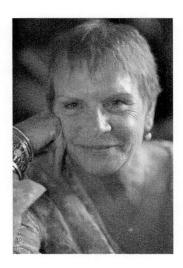

Trish Bartley has been teaching Mindfulness-Based Cognitive Therapy for Cancer in a hospital oncology center, since 2001. She has published, trained and supervised mindfulness teachers to teach this programme in many parts of the world. She has had her own personal experiences of cancer and treatment, and uses mindfulness practice to support her life and work. She is a senior teacher at the Centre for Mindfulness, Research and Practice at Bangor University, UK. She wrote *Mindfulness-Based Cognitive Therapy for Cancer* as a handbook for mindfulness-based teachers working with people with cancer.